CIOMS Guide to Vaccine Safety Communication

Report by Topic Group 3 of the CIOMS Working Group on Vaccine Safety

Council for International Organizations of Medical Sciences (CIOMS)

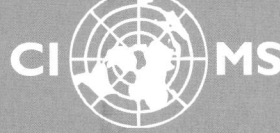

Geneva, Switzerland 2018

Copyright © 2018 by the Council for International Organizations of Medical Sciences (CIOMS)

ISBN: 978-92-9036091-9

All rights reserved. CIOMS publications may be obtained directly from CIOMS using its website e-shop module at https://cioms.ch/shop/. Further information can be obtained from CIOMS P.O. Box 2100, CH-1211 Geneva 2, Switzerland, tel.: +41 22 791 6497, www.cioms.ch, e-mail: info@cioms.ch.

CIOMS publications are also available through the World Health Organization, WHO Press, 20 Avenue Appia, CH-1211 Geneva 27, Switzerland.

Citations:
CIOMS Guide to vaccine safety communication. Report by topic group 3 of the CIOMS Working Group on Vaccine Safety. Geneva, Switzerland: Council for International Organizations of Medical Sciences (CIOMS), 2018.

Note on style:
This publication uses the World Health Organization's WHO style guide, 2nd Edition, 2013 (WHO/KMS/WHP/13.1) wherever possible for spelling, punctuation, terminology and formatting which combines British and American English conventions.

Disclaimer:
The authors alone are responsible for the views expressed in this publication and those views do not necessarily represent the decisions, policies or views of their respective institutions or companies.

Design and Layout: Paprika (Annecy, France)

ACKNOWLEDGEMENTS

The Council for International Organizations of Medical Sciences (CIOMS) gratefully acknowledges the contributions of the members of the CIOMS Working Group on Vaccine Safety (WG) who served in the topic group 3 that produced this Guide to Vaccine Safety Communication. Generous support from medicines regulatory authorities, industry, academia and other organizations and institutions provided experts and resources that facilitated the work culminating in this publication.

Each WG member and consulted reviewer participated according to their abilities and time demands as actively as they were able in the meetings and discussions, teleconference calls, email exchanges, drafting and redrafting of texts and their review, which enabled the WG and topic groups to bring the project to a successful conclusion. During the multiyear process, new members from some organizations were invited, in capacity of their expertise, to cover changes in assignments.

During the course of its work, topic group 3 evolved in its focus. Its genesis occurred at the first WG meeting in London when vaccine crisis management arose as an area needing greater public-private interaction, with Felix Arellano serving as topic group leader initially. Within the first year, his professional affiliation changed and he had to pass the baton. Ken Hartigan-Go accepted CIOMS's request to assume leadership for the topic group, broadening its scope. Following his subsequent organizational move, he passed on the lead role to Priya Bahri, who was invited by CIOMS to take charge of the topic group. Under Dr. Bahri's leadership, the topic group forged a new direction including additional member input and expanded stakeholder consultation.

Primary credit for the development, research, writing, and publication of this document goes to Priya Bahri as Editor of the Guide to Vaccine Safety Communication. CIOMS would also like acknowledge the European Medicines Agency for generously making Dr. Bahri's time available. Dr. Bahri's vision focused the topic group and through her expertise and diligent collaboration process, she brought the current Guide to fruition. Additionally, the advice and support from Patrick Zuber who heads WHO Vaccine Safety and his staff was invaluable. Karin Holm acted as the CIOMS In-House Editor throughout the process.

CIOMS appreciates the additional members of the WG who contributed at various times on the development and output of this topic group: Siti Asfijah Abdoellah, Novilia Bachtiar, Ulf Bergman, Rebecca Chandler, Peter Glen Chua, Mimi Delese Darko, Alexander Dodoo, Ken Hartigan-Go, Marie Lindquist, and Paulo Santos. Outside expertise is gratefully acknowledged from Bruce Hugman, Katrine Bach Habersaat, and Madhav Ram Balakrishnan.

During the public consultation via the CIOMS website from 28 August to 11 October 2017, comments were received from experienced institutions, namely the National Institute for Public Health and the Environment of the Netherlands, the Center of Biologics Evaluation and Research (CBER) at the US Food and Drug Administration and the World Medical Association (WMA) (see Annex 3). In addition, Heidi Larson from the London School of Hygiene and Tropical Medicine and Robert Pless from Health Canada, commented as individual experts. Their comments were welcoming and supportive to the report, and clarifications on the recommendations and updates to some of the references, as well as additions to the reading list have been implemented in to the final report in response to the comments. Unless indicated otherwise the comments from external reviewers were considered as expert, personal opinions and not necessarily representing those of their employers or affiliations. CIOMS thanks those who have commented for their time and support.

Geneva, Switzerland, December 2017

Lembit Rägo, MD, PhD
Secretary-General, CIOMS

CONTENTS

ACKNOWLEDGEMENTS III
FOREWORD VIII
ACRONYMS AND ABBREVIATIONS... IX
READER'S GUIDE X
CHAPTER 1. INTRODUCTION... 1
CHAPTER 2. CONSIDERATIONS FOR VACCINE SAFETY COMMUNICATION 7
2.1. Audiences and aims of vaccine safety communication... 7
    Figure 2.1: The social-ecological model (SEM) 8
2.2. Communicating evidence and uncertainties for informed decision-making 9
    Guidance Summary 2.2: Addressing uncertainty in vaccine safety 10
2.3. Transparency for honest communication and public trust-building 11
    Guidance Summary 2.3: Building trust in vaccine safety 11
    Example 2.3: Re-building trust in the MMR vaccine in the United Kingdom 12
2.4. Perceptions of risk as a trigger of vaccine hesitancy.. 15
    Figure 2.4: The WHO Strategic Advisory Group of Experts (SAGE) on Immunization Model of determinants of vaccine hesitancy 16
    Guidance Summary 2.4: Addressing vaccine hesitancy 18
    Example 2.4.1: Overcoming hesitancy against the MMR vaccine in sub-populations in Sweden 18
    Example 2.4.2: The need for understanding public concerns over HPV vaccines prior to licensure and launch 20

CHAPTER 3. PRODUCT LIFE-CYCLE MANAGEMENT APPROACH TO VACCINE SAFETY AND COMMUNICATION 22
3.1. Communication as part of vaccine pharmacovigilance.. 22
3.2. Pre-licensure and launch phase.. 23
    Example 3.2.1: The need for understanding concerns in different communities over the Ebola virus and vaccines prior to launching clinical trials.. 23
    Guidance Summary 3.2.1: Concept of risk management systems for medicinal products 25
    Figure 3.2: Risk management cycle 25
    Guidance Summary 3.2.2: Types of risk minimization measures for medicinal products 26
    Example 3.2.2: Risk management planning for DTPw-HBV quadrivalent vaccine.............. 26
    Example 3.2.3: The introduction of pentavalent vaccines in Kerala, India, supported by close interactions with the healthcare community and the media 27
3.3. Post-licensure phase.. 28
    Example 3.3.1: Addressing the risk of febrile seizures with a serogroup B meningococcal vaccines in the United Kingdom 29
    Example 3.3.2: Addressing the safety concern of narcolepsy for the H1N1 pandemic influenza vaccine used in Sweden 31

CHAPTER 4. VACCINE SAFETY COMMUNICATION PLANS (VACSCPS) 33
4.1. Application of a strategic communication approach to vaccine safety 33
 Figure 4.1: The P-Process of strategic health communication 33
 Checklist 4.1: Management considerations for VacSCPs 34
4.2. Developing VacSCPs on the basis of a model template 35
 Template 4.2: Template for strategic vaccine type- and situation-specific vaccine safety communication plans (VacSCPs) 36
 Guidance Summary 4.2: Developing communication strategies on vaccine benefits and risks 37
4.3. Monitoring, evaluating and maintaining VacSCPs 38
 4.3.1 Monitoring of debates and sentiments in communities and the public 39
 Example 4.3.1: Social media monitoring during polio supplementary immunization activities (SIA) in Israel 40
 Example 4.3.2: Utility of online news media monitoring for prepared communicating of the outcome of a safety assessment for HPV vaccines at the European Medicines Agency (EMA) 40

CHAPTER 5. VACCINE SAFETY COMMUNICATION SYSTEMS 42
5.1. Functions of vaccine safety communication systems 42
 Checklist 5.1: Key functions of vaccine safety communication systems 42
5.2. Multistakeholder network 42
 Table 5.2.1: Main stakeholders involved in the vaccine safety communication process 43
 Checklist 5.2: Establishing and maintaining national stakeholder networks 43
 Table 5.2.2: Purposes of multistakeholder interactions 44
 Example 5.2: Managing an adverse event following immunization with HPV vaccine in the United Kingdom 45
5.3. Regional and international awareness and collaboration 50
 Figure 5.3: Relationships of parties in global vaccine safety 50

CHAPTER 6. CAPACITY BUILDING FOR VACCINE SAFETY COMMUNICATION SYSTEMS 52
6.1. Skills and capacity requirements 52
 Checklist 6.1: Skills and capacity requirements for vaccine safety communication 52
6.2. Contents and objectives of training 53
 Table 6.2: Curriculum for vaccine safety communication 53
 Example 6.2.1: Training programme on vaccine safety communication by the WHO Regional Office for Europe (WHO-EURO) 54
 Example 6.2.2: Training resources of the Network for Education and Support in Immunisation (NESI) .. 54
6.3. Comprehensive approach to capacity building 55

ANNEX 1: READING LIST 56

ANNEX 2: CONTRIBUTION TO THE CIOMS GUIDE TO ACTIVE VACCINE SAFETY SURVEILLANCE 61

ANNEX 3: MEMBERSHIP, EXTERNAL REVIEWERS, AND MEETINGS 63

SUMMARIES & EXAMPLES

Legend:

▸ CIOMS summaries with key references in Tables grey, Checklists red, and a Template in yellow (LEVEL 1)

▸ Guidance Summaries of existing practical guidance documents with precise (linked) references blue and multicoloured Figures (LEVEL 2)

▸ Examples from real-world with references to source green (LEVEL 3)

Level 1: CIOMS Summaries

Table 5.2.1: Main stakeholders involved in the vaccine safety communication process 43

Table 5.2.2: Purposes of multistakeholder interactions 44

Table 6.2: Curriculum for vaccine safety communication... 53

Checklist 4.1: Management considerations for VacSCPs 34

Checklist 5.1: Key functions of vaccine safety communication systems...................................... 42

Checklist 5.2: Establishing and maintaining national stakeholder networks............................... 43

Checklist 6.1: Skills and capacity requirements for vaccine safety communication 52

Template 4.2: Template for strategic vaccine type- and situation-specific vaccine safety communication plans (VacSCPs).. 36

Level 2: Guidance Summaries

Guidance Summary 2.2: Addressing uncertainty in vaccine safety...10

Guidance Summary 2.3: Building trust in vaccine safety 11

Guidance Summary 2.4: Addressing vaccine hesitancy 18

Guidance Summary 3.2.1: Concept of risk management systems for medicinal products 25

Guidance Summary 3.2.2: Types of risk minimization measures for medicinal products........26

Guidance Summary 4.2: Developing communication strategies on vaccine benefits and risks 37

Figures

Figure 2.1: The social-ecological model (SEM) 8

Figure 2.4: The WHO Strategic Advisory Group of Experts (SAGE) on Immunization Model of determinants of vaccine hesitancy 16

Figure 3.2: Risk management cycle 25

Figure 4.1: The P-Process of strategic health communication 33

Figure 5.3: Relationships of parties in global vaccine safety 50

Level 3: Examples

Example 2.3: Re-building trust in the MMR vaccine in the United Kingdom 12

Example 2.4.1: Overcoming hesitancy against the MMR vaccine in sub-populations in Sweden 18

Example 2.4.2: The need for understanding public concerns over HPV vaccines prior to licensure and launch 20

Example 3.2.1: The need for understanding concerns in different communities over the Ebola virus and vaccines prior to launching clinical trials 23

Example 3.2.2: Risk management planning for DTPw-HBV quadrivalent vaccine 26

Example 3.2.3: The introduction of pentavalent vaccines in Kerala, India, supported by close interactions with the healthcare community and the media 27

Example 3.3.1: Addressing the risk of febrile seizures with a serogroup B meningococcal vaccines in the United Kingdom 29

Example 3.3.2: Addressing the safety concern of narcolepsy for the H1N1 pandemic influenza vaccine used in Sweden 31

Example 4.3.1: Social media monitoring during polio supplementary immunization activities (SIA) in Israel 40

Example 4.3.2: Utility of online news media monitoring for prepared communicating of the outcome of a safety assessment for HPV vaccines at the European Medicines Agency (EMA) 40

Example 5.2: Managing an adverse event following immunization with HPV vaccine in the United Kingdom 45

Example 6.2.1: Training programme on vaccine safety communication by the WHO Regional Office for Europe (WHO-EURO) 54

Example 6.2.2: Training resources of the Network for Education and Support in Immunisation (NESI) 54

FOREWORD

Since its inception in 1949 by the World Health Organization and UNESCO, the Council for International Organizations of Medical Sciences (CIOMS) has contributed in various roles by taking up scientific topics benefiting from collaboration across the sectors of public health agencies, medicines regulatory or competent authorities, the pharmaceutical industry, and academia. Over the years CIOMS has evolved into an independent, non-governmental international organization that provides a neutral and objective forum conducive to public-private interaction on issues concerning medical sciences, most recently focused around pharmacovigilance and bioethics.

In 2013 a new working group was formed, the CIOMS Working Group on Vaccine Safety (WG) to address unmet needs in the area of vaccine pharmacovigilance and specifically address Objective #8 of WHO's Global Vaccine Safety Initiative regarding public-private information exchange. The WG's report issued at the beginning of 2017, CIOMS Guide to Active Vaccine Safety Surveillance (Guide AVSS)[1], offers a practical step-by-step approach and a graphic algorithm to aid immunization professionals and decision-makers in determining the best course of action when confronting such challenges. The Guide AVSS provides a structured process, a checklist for evaluating the extent of data resources, and several case studies for review.

This current CIOMS Guide to Vaccine Safety Communication (Guide or report) stemmed from topic group 3 of the WG which brought together, in a unique forum, pharmacovigilance specialists and other experts from regulatory and public health authorities, the World Health Organization, and academia as well as manufacturers in emerging and industrialized countries. The Guide presents recommendations for vaccine safety communication with a specific focus on regulatory bodies. A number of communication guidance documents already exist for immunization programmes covering how to manage communication when an adverse event occurs. Few have thus far been issued addressing the specific needs of regulatory bodies or competent authorities — whether they be established authorities in high-income countries or developing authorities in resource-limited countries. Little has been published for these groups in relation to communication about risks, uncertainties, safety and safe use of the vaccine products they license.

This CIOMS report aims to fill this gap. Although the Guide sources from existing guidance documents, it compiles recommendations relevant from a regulatory perspective and creates a common ground in a way that has not been achieved otherwise at global level. The Guide stresses the fundamental importance of regulatory bodies having a system in place with skilled persons who can efficiently run vaccine safety communication in collaboration with stakeholders.

---

[1] Council for International Organizations of Medical Sciences (CIOMS). CIOMS Guide to Active Vaccine Safety Surveillance (report of the CIOMS Working Group on Vaccine Safety). Geneva: CIOMS, 2017.

ACRONYMS AND ABBREVIATIONS

AEFI	Adverse event following immunization
AVSS	Active vaccine safety surveillance
CIOMS	Council for International Organizations of Medical Sciences
ECDC	European Centre for Disease Prevention and Control
EMA	European Medicines Agency
GACVS	Global Advisory Committee on Vaccine Safety
GVSI	Global Vaccine Safety Initiative
H1N1	A pandemic flu strain
HCP	Healthcare professionals
HPV	Human papillomavirus
KAP	Knowledge, attitudes, practices
MMR	Measles mumps rubella
NGO	Non-governmental organization
NIP	National immunization program
NRA	National regulatory authority
PV	Pharmacovigilance
RLC	Resource-limited country
SAGE	Strategic Advisory Group of Experts
SEM	Social-Ecological Model
SIA	Supplementary immunization activity
TIP	Tailoring Immunization Programmes
UMC	Uppsala Monitoring Centre
UNICEF	United Nations Children's Fund
USFDA	United States Food and Drug Administration
VacSCP	Vaccine safety communication plan
VSC	Vaccine safety communication
VSN	Vaccine Safety Net
WHO	World Health Organization

READER'S GUIDE

The CIOMS Guide to Vaccine Safety Communication (Guide or report) provides an overview of strategic communication issues faced by regulators, those responsible for vaccination policies and programmes and other stakeholders involved in introducing: (1) newly-developed vaccines for the first time to market or (2) current or underutilized vaccines into new countries, regions, or populations.

The Guide discusses the complexity of vaccine safety communication (see Chapter 2) and builds upon already existing expert recommendations to fill a specific niche that is meant to be particularly useful to regulatory authorities in resource-limited countries (RLCs). The Guide draws upon recommendations from numerous institutional materials for compilation of guidance, for example, on aims (see §2.1), key functions (see §5.1), networks (see §5.2 and §5.3) and capacity-building (see Chapter 6). Where existing recommendations have been summarized, this has been done in a very condensed manner. The references provided allow for returning to the source documents for more in-depth reading on the concepts and their background if required.

Recognizing the successful implementation of strategic communication for some objectives in other areas of health, the recommendations in the Guide are based on this strategic process. However this report is not a process guide, as such processes can be adapted for the specific needs of individual regulatory bodies from general sources on health communication.

More practically and immediately tangible, the Guide presents the CIOMS template of a vaccine safety communication plan (VacSCP) to provide for proactive, prepared and responsive communication. The template allows for specific planning, monitoring and adapting of communications for each vaccine type in the given local situation (see CIOMS VacSCP Template §4.2). This is important as public sentiments differ locally by vaccine type, disease epidemiology and public debate.

As this report supports regulatory bodies, it discusses how assessment for licensure, pharmacovigilance and communication should be interactive processes within these bodies (see Chapter 3). It also considers the context regulators have to keep awareness of - in particular tensions between evidence and uncertainty, public trust and mistrust, and vaccine acceptance and vaccine hesitancy (see §2.2 and §2.4), all subject to sudden or slow change over time. It may be most appropriate for a regulatory body to build up their vaccine safety communication system and VacSCPs gradually over time in accordance with local needs.

The recommendations in this report are not only based on existing guidance, but also on established practices, experiences of immunization programmes and regulatory bodies as well as evidence from relevant research. All references are provided in footnotes. Where recommendations and considerations are not referenced, these constitute the views of the CIOMS topic group.

The Guide can be read in many ways. Of course, it can be read from beginning to end to follow its primary logic - that is, from aims and context, over pharmacovigilance and communication planning, to building up the necessary communication system. Readers may however use any section as entry point, depending on one's background and most immediate interest. Cross-references to the other sections (with hyperlinks in the digital version) are provided throughout the report allowing for flexible reading. Nonetheless Chapter 1's introduction and overview will be a suitable section with which to start upfront for all readers to understand the underlying approach of the Guide. The report also presents a number of examples of successful communication interventions around the globe to illustrate the recommendations (highlighted in green). These examples can also be read first to enter the report through gaining an initial practical understanding of the recommendations.

An additional reading list can be found in Annex I, organized by topics, guides readers for further learning and training.

CHAPTER 1.
INTRODUCTION

Vaccines transformed global health and continue to yield health gains in this century. Through improving health, immunization promises further benefits for individuals and societies at large, increasing earning power and saving healthcare costs. The range of vaccines and diseases they can prevent is expanding. Consequently, the need for strong safety surveillance of vaccine products and clear communication to inform the public is growing as well.

The World Health Organization launched the Global Vaccine Action Plan (GVAP) in 2012 for the period through 2020.[2] The GVAP is a roadmap setting targets for each vaccine-preventable disease and addressing how to bestow the full benefits of immunization to all people. Important GVAP goals are to add polio to the list of globally eradiated diseases (to join smallpox) and to accelerate progress towards the elimination of measles, rubella and neonatal tetanus. Priorities include the additional control of diseases that can be addressed through improving coverage rates of existing routine immunizations (e.g. diphtheria, Haemophilus influenzae type B (Hib), hepatitis B virus, pertussis, rubella, tetanus, and tuberculosis), and the development and use of new vaccines. The Strategic Advisory Group of Experts (SAGE) on Immunization to WHO recently produced an Assessment Report of GVAP and advised that post-2020, "the challenge will be to ensure that these gains are protected and further extended – to ensure more vaccines reach more people more rapidly."[3] This could involve countries and stakeholders directing more resources towards:[4]

1. recently developed and/or underutilized vaccines (e.g. humanpapilloma virus (HPV), pneumococcal, and rotavirus);
2. vaccines intended for regionally prevalent diseases (e.g. cholera, Japanese encephalitis, meningitis A, seasonal influenza, and yellow fever); as well as
3. new vaccines in development or on the horizon (e.g. against dengue, Ebola, or Zika viruses, human immunodeficiency virus (HIV), malaria, sexually-transmitted diseases, or an improved vaccine against tuberculosis).

The Council for International Organizations of Medical Sciences (CIOMS) can make an important contribution to meeting this challenge as one of its major aims is: "contributing to harmonised views of international systems and terminologies used for the safety surveillance of medicinal products and vaccines between stakeholders." The independent status of CIOMS has permitted the organization over the decades of its existence to facilitate the collaborations and expertise of senior scientists from national medicines regulatory authorities, academia, public health agencies, representative bodies of medical specialties and research-based biopharmaceutical companies. CIOMS has convened numerous working groups on pharmacovigilance topics, including one that produced the CIOMS report on Definition and Application of Terms for Vaccine Pharmacovigilance and an annex on Vaccines in the CIOMS IX report on Practical Approaches to Risk Minimisation for Medicinal Products.[5]

---

[2] WHO Global vaccine action plan 2011-2020
http://www.who.int/immunization/global_vaccine_action_plan/GVAP_Guiding_Principles_Measures_of_Success_and_Goals.pdf?ua=1.

[3] 2017 Assessment Report of the Global Vaccine Action Plan Strategic Advisory Group of Experts on Immunization. Geneva: World Health Organization; 2017. Licence: CC BYNC-SA 3.0 IGO, p.28

[4] SAGE meeting reports available at www.who.int/immunization/sage/meetings/2017/october/en/, accessed October 2017.

[5] CIOMS website, https://cioms.ch/about/

The Working Group's mandate, aim and addresses

To continue this work, the CIOMS Working Group on Vaccine Safety (WG) was formed to support the World Health Organization (WHO) in the implementation of the strategic objective 8 of its Blueprint of the Global Vaccine Safety Initiative (GVSI)[6], which is: "to put in place systems for appropriate interaction between national governments, multilateral agencies[7] and manufacturers at national, regional and international levels" particularly concerning underutilized and new vaccines expected to be of global, regional or local significance in the near- to long-term.

The WG divided itself into three key areas affecting vaccine safety when a newly-developed vaccine or new-to-the-country vaccine is introduced into a population. Topic group1 focused on examining the safety baseline data needed by country regulatory authorities and immunization programmes and contributed the Appendix I: Essential Vaccine Information (EVI) to the CIOMS Guide to Active Vaccine Safety Surveillance (Guide AVSS). Topic group 2 took charge of contributing the main body of the Guide AVSS. Topic group 3 concentrated on the communications aspect of vaccine safety.

Through the course of multistakeholder discussion and collaboration, over several meetings topic group 3 determined its critical value would be to create this CIOMS Guide to Vaccine Safety Communication (referred to as Guide or report) which complements other helpful documents from WHO and other organizations by filling a gap for regulatory needs applicable globally. The Guide additionally supports the implementation of strategic objective 3 of the GVSI Blueprint, which is "to develop vaccine safety communication plans at country level, to promote awareness of vaccine risks and benefits, understand the perception of the risk and prepare for managing any adverse events and concerns about vaccine safety promptly." Therefore this report is addressed particularly to the authorities in charge of vaccine pharmacovigilance at country level – usually the national regulatory authorities.

While this report addresses regulatory bodies and supports WHO's GVSI, the recommendations are also applicable to vaccine safety communication in general. In particular, national immunization programmes or other groups which may exist in some countries, have a major responsibility for programme implementation and delivery, assuming an important role relative to vaccine safety and communication. While they may have specific guidance documents available, the approach taken in this report might prove informative for them. In addition, vaccine manufacturers might learn from this report a new perspective about safety communication systems to improve their corporate pharmacovigilance systems and product-related communication interventions, facilitating interactions with their medical information and public relation functions internally, and with governmental bodies externally.

Background of existing guidance documents and approach taken by the Working Group

A number of vaccine communication guides already exist (and were reviewed by the topic group), but these are often field-oriented and primarily provide for those in charge of immunization programmes, covering in particular how to be prepared and manage communication when an adverse event occurs. Some also include guidance for healthcare professionals. So far, only a few regulatory bodies have issued guidance addressing the specific needs of regulators in relation to

---

[6] World Health Organization (WHO). Global Vaccine Safety Blueprint (WHO/IVB 12.07). Geneva: WHO, 2012. Accessible at: http://extranet.who.int/iris/restricted/bitstream/10665/70919/1/WHO_IVB_12.07_eng.pdf?ua=1.

[7] Agencies formed by several countries to serve them, such as UN system and other regional and sub-regional organizations.

communicating about risks, uncertainties, safety and safe use of the vaccine products they license (e.g. European Medicines Agency[8]).

Effective communication of assessment outcomes is, however, an important part of the mandate of regulatory bodies and expected by the public and all stakeholders, at the time a vaccine product is newly launched in a country as well as if a concern emerges later in the product life-cycle. Although this report sources from existing guidance documents, in particular those for immunization programmes, it compiles recommendations relevant from a regulatory perspective and creates a common ground in a way that has not been achieved otherwise at global level.

The existing guidance documents have been selected as references for their respective focus on certain elements of communication and the expertise they contain, reflecting current evidence and authority. They have mainly been issued by major organizations, like WHO and national and regional public health agencies, such as the Centers for Disease Control and Prevention (CDC) in the United States and the European Centre for Disease Prevention and Control (ECDC) in the European Union.

These organizational references have been complemented by publications in scientific journals on specific aspects of communication. The recommendations in this report are also based on established practices, experiences of immunization programmes and regulatory bodies, as well as evidence from relevant research and duly cited in footnotes.

Where recommendations and considerations are not referenced, these constitute the views of the CIOMS topic group.

Overall, topic group 3 dedicated itself to issue a 'guide', which means to provide recommendations based on established principles, research evidence and example-based learning. As with recommendations for any complex intervention in highly variable and continuously changing situations, the recommendations cannot be specific. Therefore this Guide is intended to provide primarily to regulators, but also to other relevant parties in charge of vaccination programmes on the country level, a foundation for understanding complex communication issues related to vaccines safety. In addition, it aims to provide general recommendations on how to create vaccine safety communication plans and deliver in real life situations high quality communication input messages for those actually in charge of the communications.

The strategic approach to communication

As some major health objectives – for example, the prevention of infection with human immunodeficiency virus (HIV) – have been achieved with support of strategic communication, the recommendations in the current Guide are based on this strategic process. However this report is not a process guide detailing who has to do what, when, why and how, as such processes can (and should) be adapted for the specifics of individual regulatory bodies from general sources on health communication.

---

[8] European Medicines Agency (EMA) and Heads of Medicines Agencies. Guideline on good pharmacovigilance practices – product- or population-specific considerations I: vaccines for prophylaxis against infectious diseases. London: EMA, 12 December 2013. Accessible at: http://www.ema.europa.eu/ema/index.jsp?curl=pages/regulation/document_listing/document_listing_000345.jsp&mid=WC0b01ac058058f32c.

The concept of communication plans

More practically and immediately tangible, this report presents the CIOMS template of a vaccine safety communication plan (VacSCP) that allows for specific planning, monitoring and adapting of communication that is proactive, prepared and responsive.

Topic group 3 of the CIOMS Working Group on Vaccine Safety proposes to define vaccine safety communication plans at country level as "individual vaccine safety communication plans that are specific to vaccine types and the local situation" (VacSCPs, see Chapter 4).

These VacSCPs need to be kept up-to-date in accordance with changing evidence and information on the quality and safety of vaccine products and their effectiveness. VacSCPs should be periodically adapted to the context of evolving public health needs and the evolving debates at policy level and in the public domain.

As regulators monitor the benefit-risk balance of the vaccines they license, they should ideally also monitor the public debate and possible rumours about vaccines in the communities and the media. For regulatory communication to be most effective, their communication plans and messages can address concerns raised by the public and fill information needs. It is understood that the individual VacSCPs may have generic elements in common or even be part of a single planning framework at country level, or that there will be local prioritization concerning which vaccines need a communication plan.

In any case, the VacSCPs are meant to focus on the safety of vaccine products as assessed by the applicable regulatory authority and do not opine on immunization policy, which falls under the responsibility of the public health authorities. The information provided by regulatory bodies needs, however, to be useful to others for making decisions on immunization programmes and immunizations of individuals. This requires listening to stakeholders as part of the communication process, in order to understand which concerns and information needs have to be addressed by regulators responsible for vaccine safety.

Overall, vaccine safety communication consists of complex processes of listening and messaging between the regulatory bodies and all stakeholders, including the manufacturers responsible for vaccine safety, the multiple institutional parties involved in immunization, the media, and most importantly, the communities and the people who should benefit from vaccines.

The concept of a systems approach to vaccine safety communication

As health and information needs are evolving, VacSCPs cannot be static plans. Therefore the topic group has taken the view that in order to manage vaccine safety communication professionally and to a high quality standard, a system is needed at the level of regulatory bodies for developing, updating, implementing and evaluating these plans. Such vaccine safety communication systems should operate continuously and always be designed for proactivity, preparedness and responsiveness. It is recommended to put a system in place with dedicated people and resources with defined objectives, functions and expertise (see §5.1). Capacity-building in this respect is very important (see Chapter 6).

This report provides added value by presenting a "systems approach" with an integration of communication as part of pharmacovigilance and risk management for vaccine products (see Chapter 3). In this respect, it is stressed that communication, no matter how skilful and carefully designed, cannot and is not meant to disguise any lack of evidence, uncertainty or flaws in the processes of safety surveillance, risk management or regulatory decision-making. The link between communication and transparency is vital (see §2.3).

In order to understand each given situation and to design effective communication interventions, it is necessary to build relationships with representatives of all stakeholders. This requires, as part of the communication system, establishment and maintenance of local and global stakeholder networks, underpinned by policies that prevent undue influences (see §5.2 and §5.3).

Contextual considerations

Of course, those engaged in vaccine safety communication cannot ignore the contexts in which they work. While vaccines have been one of the most successful health interventions and vast population groups agree with immunization,[9] at the same time there is a debate in the public domain around vaccine benefits, risks and uncertainties, and some groups and individuals are hesitant or reject vaccines, or develop mistrust in scientists and officials (see §2.4) and collaborating with stakeholders is therefore vital (see §2.3).

The systems and planning approach referenced in this Guide is considered the best way to manage communication in the event of a public health emergency, such as a pandemic, and to prevent or manage situations of crisis, which can be triggered, for example, by a public reaction to a safety concern.

Global scope of the report

Established authorities in both high-income countries and resource-limited countries (RLCs) share interests and concerns around good communication on vaccine safety, and seek approaches for improvement. The recommendations of this report are therefore valid for any country, but specific consideration has been given to resource limitations in many countries. The components for a vaccine safety communication system are presented with a view to building them up gradually, taking into account local resources, opportunities and priorities. In this way, a tailored system can be built over time.

Global sharing of examples and experience

Examples illustrating aspects of successful communication interventions and underpinning the recommendations are taken from different countries around the globe to demonstrate feasibility and value. Some examples specifically show how they can be implemented in RLCs.

The topic group deliberately did not include examples of unsuccessful communication, because rarely one has all the information to judge a specific situation, and it was also not within the scope of the topic group to engage with those responsible for communication in such cases for in-depth reviews and lessons learnt. Preference was therefore given to positive examples of successful communication to stay within a constructive spirit.

---

[9] "Immunization" as used in this report means the usage of a vaccine for the purpose of immunizing individuals. It is generally acknowledged that (1) "immunization" is a broader term than "vaccination", including active and passive immunization, and (2) immunization when used strictly implies an immune response. In keeping with other key published literature in the field of immunization, the terms "immunization" and "vaccination" are generally used interchangeably in the current report. (see Council for International Organizations of Medical Sciences (CIOMS). Definition and application of terms of vaccine pharmacovigilance (report of CIOMS/WHO Working Group on Vaccine Pharmacovigilance). Geneva: CIOMS,2012). Accessible at: https://cioms.ch/shop/product/definitions-and-applications-of-terms-for-vaccine-pharmacovigilance/.

Relationship of this report with other CIOMS reports on vaccines

This report is related to the other report of the CIOMS Working Group on Vaccine Safety, namely the CIOMS Guide to Active Vaccine Safety Surveillance (Guide AVSS).[10] Topic group 3 made a contribution to that Guide AVSS (see Annex 2 for description), given that active safety surveillance and communication are processes running in parallel and should be integrated via pharmacovigilance systems (see Chapter 3).

This report is also related to the CIOMS Definition and Application of Terms for Vaccine Pharmacovigilance, from where it draws the concept of vaccine pharmacovigilance and agreed terminology.[11]

It does not include the reporting or identifying of individual adverse events following immunization (AEFIs)[12], which can be considered as a type of communication, but for which specific guidance exists.[13]

Applicability of this report to medicines beyond vaccines

While developing the report, reviewed documents included those not specific to vaccines, but more broadly to communication about medicinal products by regulatory bodies.[14, 15, 16, 17]

Therefore, CIOMS would like to make regulatory bodies aware that the recommendations in this report could be leveraged for use in their communication systems and processes for medicines other than vaccines. The same principles, systems approach, communication plan template and related processes proposed for vaccines could be applied and tailored to other medicinal product classes, as each class will have its specific challenges in communicating for understanding, informed choice, safe and trusted use as well as adherence. There are currently few guidance documents available for other medicinal product classes of similar content combining concepts and examples, although general guides exist.[18]

---

[10] Council for International Organizations of Medical Sciences (CIOMS). CIOMS Guide to Active Vaccine Safety Surveillance (report of the CIOMS Working Group on Vaccine Safety). Geneva: CIOMS, 2017.

[11] Council for International Organizations of Medical Sciences (CIOMS). Definition and application of terms of vaccine pharmacovigilance (report of CIOMS/WHO Working Group on Vaccine Pharmacovigilance). Geneva: CIOMS, 2012). Accessible at https://cioms.ch/shop/product/definitions-and-applications-of-terms-for-vaccine-pharmacovigilance/.

[12] An adverse event following immunization (AEFI) has been defined as any untoward medical occurrence which follows immunization and which does not necessarily have a causal relationship with the usage of the vaccine. The adverse event may be any unfavourable or unintended sign, abnormal laboratory finding, symptom or disease. AEFIs can be distinguished by cause as vaccine product-related reactions, vaccine quality-related reaction, immunization error-related reaction, immunization anxiety-related reaction or be coincidental events. (see Council for International Organizations of Medical Sciences (CIOMS). Definition and application of terms of vaccine pharmacovigilance (report of CIOMS/WHO Working Group on Vaccine Pharmacovigilance). Geneva: CIOMS,2012.

[13] World Health Organization (WHO): Global Manual on Surveillance of Adverse Events Following Immunization. WHO Western Pacific Regional Office, 2012.

[14] Minister of Health Canada. Strategic risk communications framework for Health Canada and the Public Health Agency of Canada. Ottawa: Minister of Health Canada, 2007. Accessible at: https://www.canada.ca/en/health-canada/corporate/about-health-canada/activities-responsibilities/risk-communications.html.

[15] Fischhoff B, Brewer NT, Downs JS. Communicating risks and benefits: an evidence-based user's guide. Silver Spring, MD: US Food and Drug Administration, 2009.

[16] Bahri P. Public pharmacovigilance communication: a process calling for evidence-based, objective-driven strategies. Drug Saf. 2010, 33: 1065-1079.

[17] European Medicines Agency (EMA) and Heads of Medicines Agencies. Guideline on good pharmacovigilance practices (GVP) – Annex II – Templates: Communication Plan for Direct Healthcare Professional Communication (CP DHPC) Rev 1. London: EMA, 12 October 2017. Accessible at: http://www.ema.europa.eu/ema/index.jsp?curl=pages/regulation/document_listing/document_listing_000345.jsp&mid=WC0b01ac058058f32c.

[18] Communicating Risks and Benefits: An Evidence-Based User's Guide. Published by the Food and Drug Administration (FDA), US Department of Health and Human Services, August 2011. Available on FDA's Web site at http://www.fda.gov/ScienceResearch/SpecialTopics/RiskCommunication/ default.htm

CHAPTER 2.
CONSIDERATIONS FOR VACCINE SAFETY COMMUNICATION

Those engaged in vaccine safety communication need to have a clear understanding of their mandates, audiences and aims (see §2.1) and cannot ignore changing contexts in which they operate, in order to adapt for efficient achievements of the aims.

The current situation is that vaccines have been one of the most successful health interventions and vast population groups agree with immunization,[19] while at the same time there is a debate in the public domain around the benefits and risks of vaccines, in particular when a safety concern arises, and some groups and individuals are hesitant or reject vaccines (see §2.4).

The challenge for communication is to operate efficiently in a field of tension between public expectations and concerns, scientific evidence and uncertainty (see §2.2). Vaccine safety communicators must also pay careful attention to the relationship between communication, transparency and public trust (see §2.3).

2.1. Audiences and aims of vaccine safety communication

The communication discussed in this report happens between regulatory authorities responsible for the safety of vaccines as medicinal products and multiple stakeholders, including public health authorities, immunization advisory committees, ministries of health, manufacturers with their own responsibility for the safety of their vaccines, healthcare professionals in their intermediary role, and the wider public. The public consists of multiple groups, including in particular those vaccinated or for whom immunization is intended, parents, families and carers, religious, community and public opinion leaders, healthcare professionals, whether modern or traditional, as well as journalists and others active in the news or social media (see §5.3).

Those responsible for infectious disease control often use the social ecological model (SEM) as a theory-based framework for understanding the multifaceted and interactive effects of personal and environmental factors that determine the behaviours of individuals and groups.[20] Without going into detailed recommendations on how this framework could be applied to vaccine safety communication by regulatory authorities, Figure 2.1 below shows how the SEM visualizes the complex relationships between the stakeholders and provides a conceptual framework for regulators to create their own local SEM and map their interactions.

---

[19] "Immunization" as used in this report means the usage of a vaccine for the purpose of immunizing individuals. It is generally acknowledged that (1) "immunization" is a broader term than "vaccination", including active and passive immunization, and (2) immunization when used strictly implies an immune response. In keeping with other key published literature in the field of immunization, the terms "immunization" and "vaccination" are - in general - used interchangeably in the current report. (see Council for International Organizations of Medical Sciences (CIOMS). Definition and application of terms of vaccine pharmacovigilance (report of CIOMS/WHO Working Group on Vaccine Pharmacovigilance). Geneva: CIOMS, 2012). Accessible at: https://cioms.ch/shop/product/definitions-and-applications-of-terms-for-vaccine-pharmacovigilance/.

[20] United Nations Children's Fund (UNICEF). What are the Social Ecological Model (SEM), and Communication for Development (C4D)? New York: UNICEF. Accessible at: https://www.unicef.org/cbsc/files/Module_1_SEM-C4D.docx.

Figure 2.1: The social-ecological model (SEM)[21]

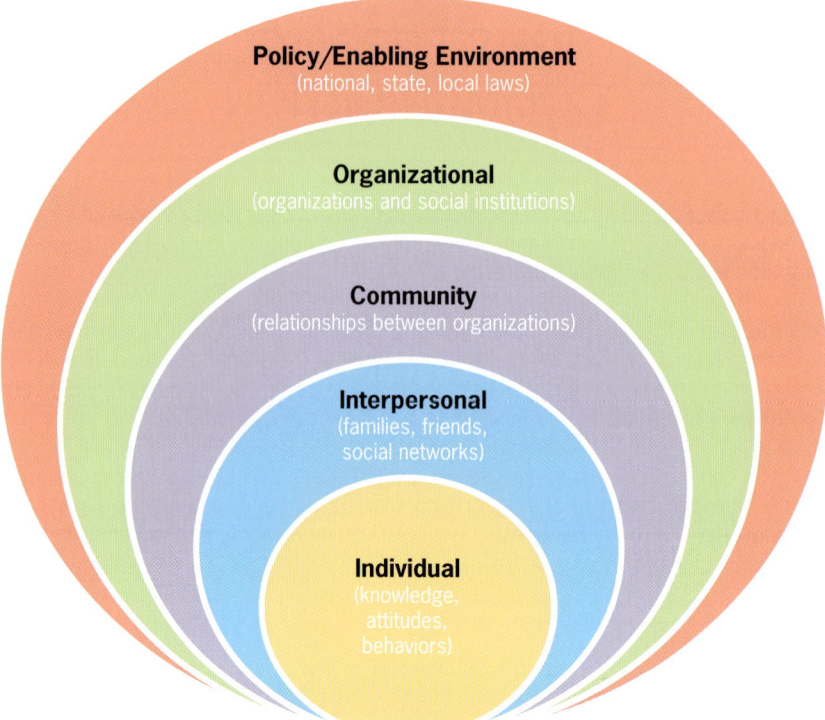

In the communication process, the roles of listening and speaking should alternate between stakeholders, who should not be viewed as opponents, but as partners in an exchange over a topic of major public interest, in order to safeguard health for individuals and as a common good. Therefore, the common language where regulators call stakeholders and especially the general public and its sub-populations 'audiences' could be misleading if that would be understood as those expected to listen without having a voice of their own. The term 'audience' is used in this report to refer to those whom vaccine safety communication systems are supposed to serve, above all the public as a whole, its sub-populations, and its individual members, healthcare professionals and health policy decision-makers.

Any party, subgroups or individuals may take particular roles in shaping knowledge, attitudes, practices (KAP) of individuals and groups, but in particular opinion leaders in healthcare, community and religious leaders, journalists, trusted governmental or nongovernmental organizations, and interest groups like anti-vaccine groups, women's groups or citizen watchdog groups. An opinion leader can also come from outside a concerned community or country.

In line with the mandate of regulatory bodies to assess and licence medicines and continuously assess and supervise medicines after licensure, regulatory vaccine safety communication with stakeholders may benefit from having the following communication aims:

---

[21] United Nations Children's Fund (UNICEF). What are the Social Ecological Model (SEM), and Communication for Development (C4D)? New York: UNICEF. Accessible at: https://www.unicef.org/cbsc/files/Module_1_SEM-C4D.docx. UNICEF adapted their model from the Centers for Disease Control and Prevention (CDC), The Social Ecological Model: A Framework for Prevention, http://www.cdc.gov/violenceprevention/overview/social-ecologicalmodel.html.

- understanding KAP and related concerns and information needs (and ideally underlying mental models)[22] of the audiences with regard to vaccines;
- providing accurate and full information about the safety profiles and benefit-risk balances of vaccine products for supporting informed choice of individuals and policy-makers in relation to immunization;
- demonstrating trustworthiness of the vaccine safety surveillance system (pharmacovigilance) for trust-building; and
- preventing and managing crisis situations due to safety concerns over vaccines.

A sub-objective is to provide the information in formats that may support healthcare professionals and vaccinators when communicating with individuals, such as (potential) vaccines (people receiving vaccinations), carers and community leaders. Communication in the public domain impacts on interpersonal communication between individuals in healthcare settings, as it occurs (e.g. when discussing informed consent for study participation, proposed vaccination of children, or suspected harm due to a vaccine).

2.2. Communicating evidence and uncertainties for informed decision-making

The issue of the general individual freedom of choice in life - versus the need for certain behaviours for community good - bears potential for conflict. From a perspective of communication and increasingly shared medical decision-making[23] and community participation, the concept of informed choice about whether to vaccinate or not is widely accepted. Informed choice and the related informed consent are complex concepts and far more demanding than is often understood. There is complexity in the scientific issues and how to communicate them in a way generally understandable as well as in the psychological, political and religious factors of individuals and groups. Informed choice can arise only when the questions, doubts, preoccupations and emotional needs of individuals and groups are accurately addressed, probably over a long period of time. Even when such concerns are accurately addressed, there may still be vaccine refusal, a decision entirely within the rights of individuals in countries where the ethical principle of voluntariness is upheld. Choice will arise from a multiplicity of influences with scientific evidence maybe playing a quite minor part, but for informed choice clear communication of the evidence is essential.

Intrinsic to the scientific approach is to acknowledge that each piece of evidence is surrounded by uncertainty to some degree, depending on the robustness of the evidence. In addition evidence can also raise new questions and detect areas of missing knowledge. While the most important step is to generate evidence to reduce uncertainty in important areas, decisions will always have to be taken despite some uncertainty.

Communication for risks is therefore only complete with its evidence-base and honesty over remaining uncertainties, and should at the same time prevent undue amplification of risk perception in society. Communication interventions can clarify what is known and what is unknown, what confidence one can have in the robustness of existing knowledge and the current plausibility and relevance of potential unknown issues. Guidance on how to address uncertainty is summarized in Guidance Summary 2.2.

---

[22] A mental model corresponds to beliefs, in which knowledge, uncertainties and unknowns get merged. New information is processed within a mental model, and this process is called perception [See Morgan MG, Fischhoff B, Bostrom A, and Atman CJ. Risk communication: a mental models approach. Cambridge: Cambridge University Press, 2002. and Slovic P. The feeling of risk: new perspectives on risk perception. London, Washington DC: Earthscan, 2010.]

[23] Elwyn G, Edwards A, Thompson R. Shared decision making in health care. 3rd ed. Oxford: Oxford University Press, 2016.

Guidance Summary 2.2: Addressing uncertainty in vaccine safety

From the report on a United States Institute of Medicines (IOM) workshop dedicated to communicating uncertainty in relation to pharmaceutical products[24], principles for communicating uncertainty in relation to the safety of vaccines can be derived and adapted as follows:

- Gain clarity over the type of uncertainty such as:
  - statistical uncertainty or other methodological limitations of existing evidence,
  - uncertainty based on surrogate primary outcomes (e.g. antibody development, or, for HPV vaccines, development of genital lesions and warts as surrogate outcome for cervical cancer risk),
  - uncertainty due to novelty of the vaccine product and early stage of evidence gathering under real conditions of vaccine use, and
  - uncertainty based on limited evidence at early stage of detecting a signal of a rare potential adverse effect of a vaccine, as the type of uncertainty defines the communication content with regard to uncertainty;
- Acknowledge the dynamics of scientific evidence as well as:
  - the complexity of benefit-risk assessment
  - the decision-making processes for regulatory licensure and individual patients, including
  - the need for interpretation of available and missing data;
- Listen to views of the public and explore values of society, in order to establish:
  - principles,
  - thresholds of risk tolerance and
  - benefit-risk trade-offs for decision-making in situation of uncertainty;
- Foster transparency about:
  - robustness of evidence,
  - type of uncertainties,
  - sensitivity analysis of different possible scenarios of areas where data is missing and
  - decision-making, including about
  - how convergence is reached between experts or how divergent views have been addressed;
- Demonstrate, towards the public, commitment and quality assuring processes to achieve best possible decisions for individual and public health as the outcome of the benefit-risk assessment in situations of uncertainty and focus on thereby earning trust.

---

[24] US Institute of Medicine (IOM). Characterizing and communicating uncertainty in the assessment of benefits and risks of pharmaceutical products - workshop summary. Washington, DC: The National Academies Press, 2014.

2.3. Transparency for honest communication and public trust-building

In this respect, it is stressed that communication, no matter how skilful and carefully designed, cannot and is not meant to disguise any lack of evidence or uncertainty or flaws in the processes of safety surveillance, risk management or regulatory decision-making. The link between communication and transparency is vital.

Further, a prerequisite to the effectiveness of the communication is that the regulatory authority as the sender of information is trusted as an evidence-based, honest and credible organization known for its integrity, and that the trustworthiness of the vaccine safety surveillance (pharmacovigilance) system is well demonstrated. Guidance on how to build trust in the area of vaccine safety is provided in Guidance Summary 2.3, and is illustrated by Example 2.3.

Guidance Summary 2.3: Building trust in vaccine safety

A report of the European Centre for Disease Prevention and Control (ECDC)[25] on building trust in immunization programmes and the Vaccine Confidence Project at the London School of Hygiene & Tropical Medicine[26] has been used as the basis for the following recommendations for regulatory authorities for building trust in the area of vaccine safety:

- Engage in transparency;
- Build professional-personal relationships with all stakeholders (see §5.3) over time and specifically at local and 'grass root' level for a multistakeholder dialogue;
- Apply the stepwise communication process with monitoring of knowledge, attitudes, practices (KAP) (see §2.1) and related concerns and information needs;
- Foster the participation of all parties in the vaccine assessment and communication processes to ensure that public concerns are listened to and are taken seriously;
- Target specifically vaccine-hesitant groups (see §2.4) and those who are undecided and need information;
- Pay attention to building trust in the safety processes for the vaccines within the healthcare sector, as providers need to feel confident that they are recommending safe and effective vaccines and can confidently answer the growing questions from parents;
- Approach community, religious and political leaders and establish cooperation on vaccine matters (note that when excluded, such leaders can become barriers to public trust);
- Explain to the public how personal data accruing from these processes are protected;
- Understand barriers to trust in your environment and find solutions to overcome these barriers;
- Think beyond the vaccine and consider the historical as well as the current societal and political factors that could influence public trust;
- Communicate with the public on a new vaccine or a new vaccine safety concern proactively and continuously, in order to avoid:

---

[25] European Centre for Disease Prevention and Control (ECDC). Communication on immunisation: building trust. Stockholm: ECDC, 2012. Accessible at: http://ecdc.europa.eu/en/publications/Publications/TER-Immunisation-and-trust.pdf.

[26] London School of Hygiene & Tropical Medicine. The Vaccine Confidence Project; Accessible at: www.vaccineconfidence.org.

- information vacuums in the public domain and room for speculations and misleading rumours, and
- appearing passive and late in investigations and health protection;

▶ Be prepared for immediate communication in response to queries from the public;

▶ Be honest in providing information and do not hide uncertainties (see §2.2);

▶ Add to the key messages bridging information that can connect the new information with the mental models and KAP (see §2.1) prevalent in the public;

▶ Keep consistency between messages and explain changes and how new information links with what was known before;

▶ Monitor media debates and, in case of misinformation, provide input to debates with corrective information;

▶ When countering a negative rumour or misleading information, consider the 'fertile ground' factors that make the rumour popular in the first place and address those in addition to providing corrective information;

▶ Consider participating in the certification of the WHO's Global Advisory Committee on Vaccine Safety (GACVS) website: Vaccine Safety Net portal for websites that provide information on vaccine safety and adhere to good information practices (http://www.vaccinesafetynet.org/);[27]

▶ Always be non-judgmental and do not dismiss public concerns because they are based on belief instead of evidence. Where religious beliefs are involved, find ways to make vaccines acceptable within the given religious belief;

▶ When engaging and communicating with the public, be respectful and express commitment through the tone of messages.

Specific guidance on partnering with religious leaders and groups has been made available by UNICEF.[28]

Example 2.3: Re-building trust in the MMR vaccine in the United Kingdom

Starting in 1996, a group based at the Royal Free Hospital, London, United Kingdom (UK) published a series of articles in scientific journals that purported to show variously that measles virus, measles vaccine and measles-mumps –rubella (MMR) vaccine were respectively associated with inflammatory bowel disease and autism. Despite the lack of any credible evidence linking the measles virus and measles vaccine with bowel disease, nor the MMR vaccine with bowel disease and autism, the single measles vaccine was advised by health officials as an alternative. Despite these fundamental illogicalities, each pronouncement was given considerable media credibility supported by parents and lawyers who were seeking compensation.

---

[27] World Health Organization (WHO). Vaccine safety net. Accessible at: http://www.who.int/vaccine_safety/initiative/communication/network/vaccine_safety_websites/en/.

[28] United Nations Children's Fund (UNICEF). Building trust in immunization: partnering with religious leaders and groups. New York: UNICEF; 2004. Available at: https://www.unicef.org/publications/index_20944.html.

MMR jab 'may cause autism'

The consequence was rapid erosion of trust in the safety of MMR by parents and healthcare professionals. Before the onset of fears over MMR vaccine safety, vaccine coverage had been more than 90% by the second birthday. Measles had been eliminated from the UK. Coverage fell progressively to a national average of less than 80% with coverage of less than 70% in some localities, especially in London. Small outbreaks of measles were restricted by the previous high population immunity. Much research amongst parents showed that whilst they were concerned about the safety of MMR, they were not concerned about the potential seriousness of measles.

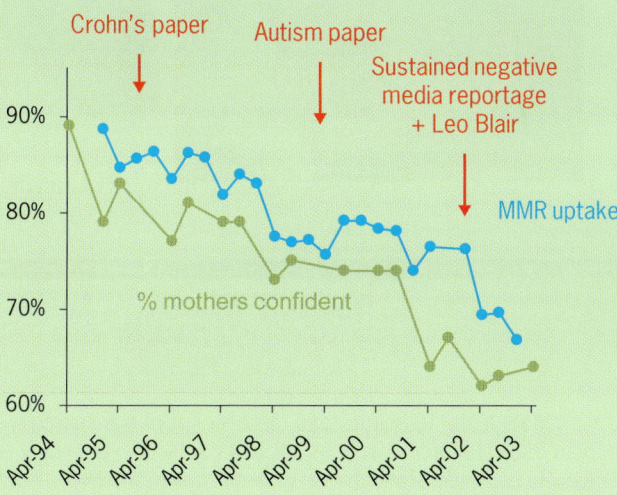

MMR uptake at 16 months and proportion of mothers believing in complete or almost complete safety of MMR vaccine

Source: graphic provided with permission by Davis Salisbury, Global Health Security, Chatham House, London.[29]

---

[29] David Salisbury, Centre for Global Health Security, Chatham House, London UK, through email 12 Feb 2016 provided as a PowerPoint slide in document, with reference to presentation by Jo Yarwood, UK Department of Health, Public Health England, 23 October 2012. Yarwood credits on slide 15: Thanks to Prof. Brent Taylor, Community Child Health at the Royal Free and University College Medical School, London, https://www.slideshare.net/meningitis/jo-yarwood-informing-the-public-about-immunisation.

Such interpretation was entirely rational in the face of repeated media reports raising fears over the MMR vaccine and autism and in the light of measles having been eliminated. Research also showed that the most trusted sources of health advice were local providers – general practitioners, practice nurses and health visitors. The UK Department of Health's communication strategy was built therefore on ensuring that those providing advice had the best information readily available to give to parents and to ensure that parents could also easily access sources of trustworthy material. For the former, a suite of materials was developed and tested that addressed concerns from the least to the most literate, readily available in hard copy or online, for the latter. The website "MMR - The Facts"[30] was accessed frequently. It was updated whenever new information became available and was much valued by parents and journalists.

Probably, the most telling event in the turnaround of opinion was the work of the investigative journalist, Brian Deer. His reports, and website, revealed much of the hitherto unknown background of the research probity leading to an investigation by the UK General Medical Council with the consequence of the removal of the licence to practice of the lead protagonist on the grounds of serious professional misconduct, including 'acting dishonestly and irresponsibly.' From this point onwards, public opinion and indeed the reporting by journalists changed considerably.

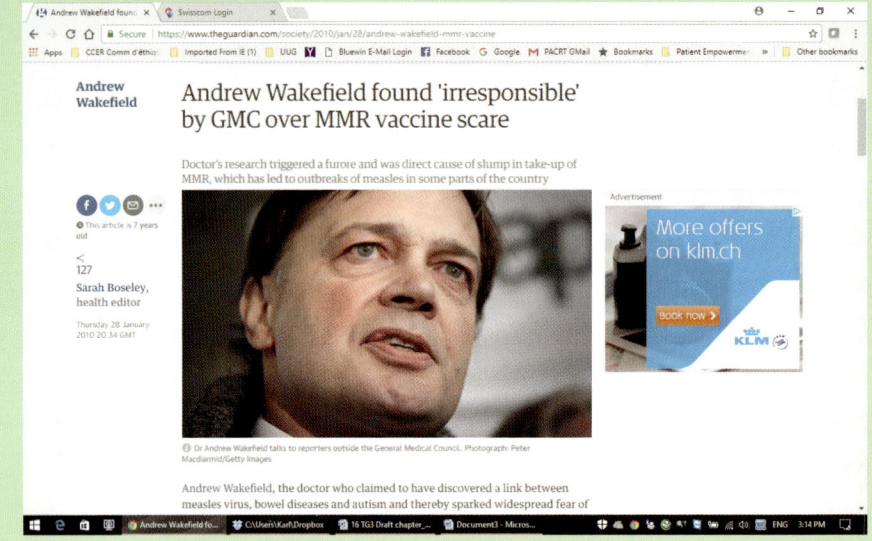

MMR vaccine coverage has quietly and consistently risen to its present levels – back over 90%.[31]

For communication, it is fundamental to understand the concept of transparency.
Transparency refers to an organization's openness about its activities, providing reliable and timely information that is accessible and understandable on what it is doing, where and how its activities take place, and how the organization is performing, unless the information is deemed confidential.[32] This should include conflict of interest declarations of those involved in assessment and decision-making

---

[30] UK Government Web Archive. NHS Immunisation Information. The Science and history of immunisation and about the vaccines in the routine UK immunisation schedule. MMR The Facts. Archived on 5 Jul 2009 http://webarchive.nationalarchives.gov.uk/20090705184233/ http://www.immunisation.nhs.uk/Vaccines/MMR

[31] Example provided by David Salisbury, Centre for Global Health Security, Chatham House, London, United Kingdom.

[32] World Health Organization (WHO). WHO accountability framework. Geneva: WHO, 2015.

as well as documentation how these are managed to avoid partiality, bias and perceptions of undue commercial influence.[33]

While both communication and transparency processes make information available to the public, they are distinguished by their objectives: transparency serves accountability over decision-making; communication aims at behaviours[34] - here the informed and safe vaccination behaviours. Communication and transparency are however linked, because transparency of the communicating organization demonstrates its trustworthiness - provided it meets the expected standards for vaccine assessment - and this makes the communication more effective.[35]

In the area of vaccine safety, transparency of regulatory authorities should make information, such as assessment reports and meeting minutes, available to the public, as much as possible proactively and otherwise upon request. This will allow the public to better understand the data gathering process, as well as the licensing, risk assessment and decision-making processes in which stakeholders are involved. By being transparent, authorities can clarify a situation to the public, acknowledge their concerns and provide relevant information about issues where the public has limited knowledge.[36] Policies need to be in place to assure confidentiality of personal data and the quality of the documents made available to the public.

2.4. Perceptions of risk as a trigger of vaccine hesitancy

Vaccine hesitancy is seen in low, middle and high-income countries around the globe. The term refers to delaying acceptance of or refusing vaccines that are on offer. Vaccine hesitancy is complex and situation-specific, varying across time, place and vaccine products.[37] Although the term vaccine hesitancy has been widely adopted to describe behaviour critical of or hostile to vaccination, it is a catch-all category rather than a coherent concept.[38] It presumes to cover a very wide range of attitudes and behaviours, influenced by multiple and differential causes and sources, both within individuals and across populations. It seems to imply an unspecified point on a spectrum from extreme opposition to full acceptance, a point which may not represent truly the entire position of an individual or society as a whole. It does not, for example, easily include at the same time the knowledgeable, vaccine-favouring individual or parent who has questions or doubts about a specific vaccine, the parent critically opposed to all vaccines and the generally ill-informed or difficult-to-reach parent whose children are not brought forward for immunization. For the time being, however, this report refers to the term vaccine hesitancy as a shortcut for this range of underlying knowledge, attitudes, practices (KAP) and related concerns and information needs.

Vaccine hesitancy arises in a complex matrix of events and influences, including the proliferation of news and social media as well as website of organizations in the internet, reliable or dubious,

---

[33] European Centre for Disease Prevention and Control (ECDC). Communication on immunisation: building trust. Stockholm: ECDC; 2012. Accessible at: http://ecdc.europa.eu/en/publications/Publications/TER-Immunisation-and-trust.pdf.

[34] Bahri P. Public pharmacovigilance communication: a process calling for evidence-based, objective-driven strategies. Drug Saf. 2010, 33: 1065-1079.

[35] Slovic P. Perceived risk, trust and democracy. In: Cvetkovich G, Löfstedt RE, eds. Social trust and the management of risk. London: Earthscan, 1999: 42-52.

[36] European Centre for Disease Prevention and Control (ECDC). Communication on immunisation: building trust. Stockholm: ECDC; 2012. Accessible at: http://ecdc.europa.eu/en/publications/Publications/TER-Immunisation-and-trust.pdf.

[37] Larson HJ, Jarret C, Eckersberger E, Smith DM, Paterson P. Understanding vaccine hesitancy around vaccines and vaccination from a global perspective: a systematic review of published literature, 2007-2012..

[38] Peretti-Watel P, Larson HJ, Ward JK, Schulz WS, Verger P. Vaccine hesitancy: clarifying a theoretical framework for an ambiguous notion. PLOS Currents Outbreaks. 2015 Feb 25 . Edition 1.

of variable quality and often confusing or contradictory. There are many complex and wide-ranging reasons for negative sentiments towards vaccines and vaccine hesitancy (see Figure 2.4), and amongst them concerns over safety are a major reason for vaccine hesitancy.[39]

Figure 2.4: The WHO Strategic Advisory Group of Experts (SAGE) on Immunization Model of determinants of vaccine hesitancy[40]

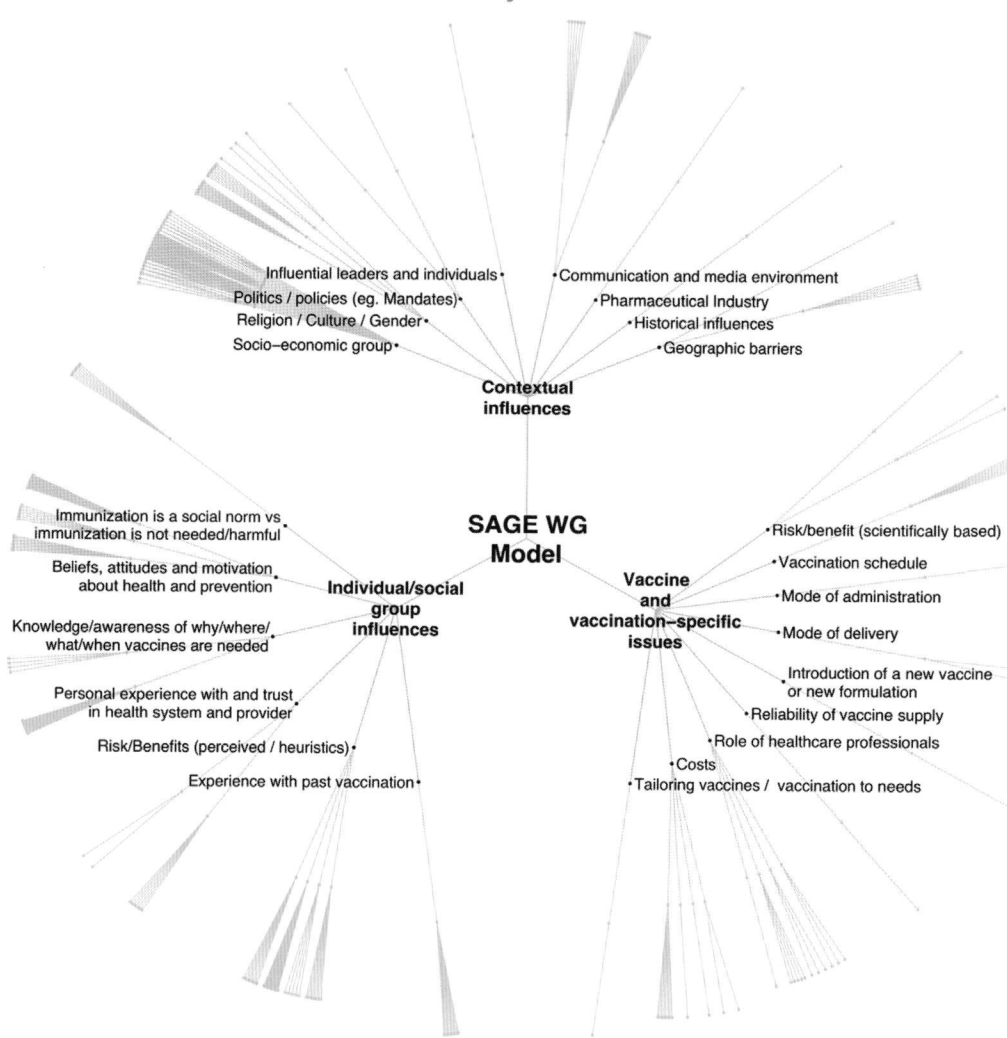

Vaccine hesitancy may however also come from a general climate of mistrust that is not specific to vaccines, but linked to lack of trust in governments, industry, or science. Among populations in resource-limited countries, some vaccine hesitancy could be related to suspicions of the motivation of donors to or foreign programme management of immunization campaigns. What is often also overlooked is that vaccine hesitancy may be understood, in some situations, as the other side of simultaneously present positive sentiments towards vaccines, i.e. expectations that they bring benefits

---

[39] Larson HJ, Jarret C, Eckersberger E, Smith DM, Paterson P. Understanding vaccine hesitancy around vaccines and vaccination from a global perspective: a systematic review of published literature, 2007-2012..

[40] Larson HJ, Jarret C, Eckersberger E, Smith DM, Paterson P, 2007-2012.

and should not harm.[41] Some argue that high expectations of vaccines may lead to heightened awareness and frustration over risks.[42]

Vaccine sentiments, acceptance and hesitancy are not static but may change as their determinants change over time or suddenly, or as a serious vaccine-preventable disease arises newly or changes in its incidence or severity, due to or independently from immunization. There is a specific potential for vaccine hesitancy when the public perception of the risk of the disease is low. In particular when diseases have become rare as the result of immunization programmes (e.g. measles, polio) and the public has little first-hand experience of the targeted diseases, perceptions of vaccine risks may be heightened in comparison to the risks of the disease. This contributes to the challenges of vaccine safety communication. On the other hand, when vaccines are perceived to be effective in preventing diseases that people are afraid of, vaccine acceptability can increase. Insufficient vaccine availability may then become an issue, prompting the need to communicate difficult decisions about prioritization of immunization target populations.

Vaccine hesitancy is not new,[43] and there are as number of examples from different parts of the world where vaccine introduction was rejected en masse by the population intended to benefit from it (e.g. the "Revolt da vacina" in Brazil in 1904[44] and HPV vaccine rejection by mothers in Romania[45]). In another example, religious or political leaders intervened in northern Nigeria[46] and Pakistan[47] to hinder the polio vaccine immunization programmes. Individual (as opposed to en masse) vaccine hesitancy, though collectively generating large numbers, appears currently to be a feature of high-income countries.

As the contexts of vaccine hesitancy vary enormously from region to region and from country to country, no comprehensive solution can be proposed. The underlying principle of any solution, however, lies in sensitive and empathic engagement and communication with individuals and communities based on an authentic understanding of the sentiments and concerns of multiple segments of the population, in particular those where doubt, resistance, mistrust or hostility is held. Comprehensive, transparent and comprehensible evidence-based safety information is a critical element of the process, but only a part. Working on trust-building is essential too (see §2.3). However, vaccine hesitancy can be addressed, and Guidance Summary 2.4 provides advice about how regulatory authorities can contribute. While reaching out to vaccine-hesitant populations falls under the remit of the public health agencies and immunization programmes, as described in Example 2.4.1, regulatory authorities can support their efforts with providing information about vaccine safety and vaccine pharmacovigilance systems (see Chapter 3). In return they can use the in-depth audience insights of the immunization programmes, in order to ensure that the information needs of all sub-audiences are fulfilled.

---

[41] Leach M, Fairhead J. Vaccine Anxieties: global science, child health and society. London: Taylor & Francis Earthscan; 2007.

[42] Leach M, Fairhead J. 2007.

[43] The College of Physicians of Philadelphia. History of anti-vaccination movements. Philadelphia, PA: The College of Physicians of Philadelphia ; 2017. Accessible at: https://www.historyofvaccines.org/content/articles/history-anti-vaccination-movements.

[44] Hochman G. Priority, Invisibility and Eradication: The History of Smallpox and the Brazilian Public Health Agenda. Medical History. 2009, 53(2):229-252.

[45] Craciun C, Baban A. Who will take the blame?: understanding the reasons why Romanian mothers declined HPV vaccination for their daughters. Vaccine. 2012; 30: 6789-6793.

[46] Ghinai I, Willott C, Dadari I, Larson HJ. Listening to the rumours: what the northern Nigeria polio vaccine boycott can tell us ten years on. Glob Public Health. 2013; 8: 1138–1150. Accessible at: https://www.ncbi.nlm.nih.gov/pmc/articles/PMC4098042/.

[47] Walsh D. Polio crisis deepens in Pakistan. New York Times. 26 Nov 2014. Accessible at: https://www.nytimes.com/2014/11/27/world/asia/gunmen-in-pakistan-kill-4-members-of-anti-polio-campaign.html?_r=0.

Guidance Summary 2.4: Addressing vaccine hesitancy

The WHO Strategic Advisory Group of Experts (SAGE) on Immunization has reviewed and identified strategies to address vaccine hesitancy. Based on these strategies,[48] the following recommendations have been formulated for regulatory authorities:

- Aim to increase knowledge and awareness surrounding vaccine safety, efficacy and quality, safe use advice and pharmacovigilance;
- Tailor the intervention to the relevant populations and their specific concerns or information gaps, including those which are discussed by vaccine-hesitant groups;
- Interact with local communities and healthcare professionals and engage with influential leaders, including religious leaders;
- Introduce education initiatives, particularly those that embed new knowledge into tangible health outcomes;
- Employ multi-component communication and follow-ups as needed.

In general, interventions that are applicable to the individual only from a distance (e.g. posters, websites, media releases, and radio announcements) have some, but usually smaller benefit than closer, personal interactions. However, the application of mass media to target parents with low levels of health service awareness still appears to have a valid place in effective communication, and there is good potential for a true positive effect across a larger population.

Example 2.4.1: Overcoming hesitancy against the MMR vaccine in sub-populations in Sweden

Two groups in the Swedish population have previously been identified as hard-to-reach for measles-mumps-rubella (MMR) immunization, based on documented low vaccination coverage: the anthroposophic community in Järna and the Somali community in Rinkeby and Tensta. The vaccination coverage among 2-year-olds in 2012 in both these communities was low (4.9% in Järna, 69.7% in Tensta and 71.5% in Rinkeby) compared to the national average of 97.2%.

Järna is a suburb south of Stockholm with a population of about 7,000 people and about 140–150 births per year. A portion of the population follows a lifestyle based upon the philosophies of Rudolf Steiner who advocated for a holistic view of health with particular views regarding food, health, and education. Many people practicing an anthroposophic way of life are hesitant towards MMR vaccination, because they believe that a measles infection is good for the child's physical and mental health development. Several outbreaks of measles and rubella have occurred in Järna and in nearby areas in recent years. In 2012, 23 cases of measles and 50 cases of rubella were reported as originating from Järna.

Rinkeby and Tensta are districts located in the northwest part of Stockholm with a high percentage of residents with foreign backgrounds, with 30% of the population of Somali origin. In 2013, the population in the Rinkeby district was 16,047 people, including 1,638 children under five years old (8.9%), and in Tensta the population was 18,866 people, including 1,673 children under five years old (10.2%). In these regions, repeated studies have revealed that Somali women in the area do not want to vaccinate their children against MMR, because they believe that the vaccine can cause autism.

---

[48] Jarret C, Wilson R, O'Leary M, Eckersberger E, Larson HJ; SAGE Working Group on Vaccine Hesitancy. Strategies for addressing vaccine hesitancy: a systematic review. Vaccine 2015; 33: 4180-4190. .

> As a response, the public health agency of Sweden used a tool developed by WHO Europe called Tailoring Immunization Programmes (TIP). The aim of TIP is to identify and increase the knowledge state about vaccines in groups with low vaccination coverage. The TIP methods are based on behavioural theories and planning models for health programmes, including social marketing and communication, with focus on behavioural change. TIP includes both an analysis method to understand the interests, characteristics and needs of different population groups and individuals in a society as well as tools to support the work of national immunization programmes with the goal of designing targeted strategies that increase acceptance of immunization.
>
> The results of the TIP analysis in Sweden revealed that communication strategies needed to be strengthened at the local and individual level in these areas with low vaccination coverage and that these interventions should be carried out for an extended period of time. Furthermore, communication with healthcare professionals was considered essential to provide them with relevant and evidence-based information about vaccines as well as about the people's attitudes toward them. Parents from the anthroposophic and Somali communities requested neutral information about the benefits and risks of vaccines and an objective dialogue with healthcare professionals. The Swedish public health agency proposed several targeted communication and education initiatives, including a peer-to-peer project, in-depth educational interventions in vaccinology for healthcare professionals and targeted information about the importance of being vaccinated with MMR before travelling abroad.
>
> In their conclusions, the public health agency noted that the project has provided a foundation and guidance for the continued work in communicating about MMR immunization. [49, 50, 51]

As vaccine hesitancy can be triggered by safety concerns, it is helpful to understand how cognitive factors impact on perceptions of risk. This understanding can also be useful for communication planning and preparedness. The cognitive and psychological decision-making sciences have identified a number of characteristics of risks, so-called cognitive factors, which may increase the perception of risk of individuals and groups. These include that a risk may be involuntary, imposed, novel, man-made, related to technology or result in a dreadful outcome, in particular after a long latency period. Other factors relate to a risk being subject to uncertainty, scientific controversy or public debate. The most powerful factors are present when a risk possibly concerns women, children, sexuality, reproduction and future generations, or is illustrated by identifiable victims and personal stories.[52]

Research has also shown that cognitive factors can lead to what is called social risk amplification, i.e. a perception of heightened risk, often triggered by debate in groups or society as a whole.[53] Where cognitive factors are present, the need for well-prepared and conducted risk communication early on prior to licensure/launch and throughout the life-cycle of a vaccine can be predicted. Example 2.4.2 demonstrates how applying these findings from risk psychology can help in prioritization efforts in

---

[49] Folkhälsomyndigheten. Barriers and motivating factors to MMR vaccination in communities with low coverage in Sweden: implementation of the WHO's Tailoring Immunization Programmes (TIP) method. Solna: Folkhälsomyndigheten,2015. Accessible under: https://www.folkhalsomyndigheten.se/pagefiles/20261/Barriers-motivating-factors-MMR-vaccination-communities-low-coverage-Sweden-15027.pdf.

[50] Byström E, Lindstrand A, Likhite N, Butler R, Emmelin M. Parental attitudes and decision-making regarding MMR vaccination in an anthroposophic community in Sweden: a qualitative study. Vaccine. 2014, 32: 6752-6757.

[51] Example provided b yChandler R, Uppsala Monitoring Centre (UMC), Sweden, confirmed through personal communication 10 February 2016.

[52] Bennett P. Understanding responses to risk: some basic findings. In: Bennett P, Calman K. Risk communication and public health. Oxford: Oxford University Press; 1999. (Quoting Fischhhoff B, Slovic P, Lichtenstein S, Read S, Coombes B. How safe is safe enough?: a psychometric study of attitudes towards technological risks and benefits. Policy Science. 1978, 9: 127-152.; Gardner GT, Gould LC. Public perceptions of risks and benefits of technology. Risk Analysis. 1989, 9: 225-242.; Slovic P. Informing and educating about risks. Risk Analysis. 1986, 6: 403-415.)

[53] Kasperson RE, Renn O, Slovic P, Brown HS, Emel J, Goble R, et al. The social amplification of risk: a conceptual framework. Risk Analysis. 1988, 8: 177-187.

the area of vaccines. While a number of cognitive factors are present in many vaccines, some are specific to certain vaccines.

Example 2.4.2: The need for understanding public concerns over HPV vaccines prior to licensure and launch

Vaccines against the human papillomavirus (HPV) were licensed as of 2006 and the public debate prior to their licensure and launch in various countries of the world demonstrates the relevance of understanding cognitive factors in vaccine safety communication, to enable addressing concerns pro-actively through risk assessment and communication.

Research has identified a number of cognitive factors that have the potential to increase risk perception in a society. These factors include relatedness of a topic to children, women, sexuality, reproduction and future generations.[54] Given the transmission of HPV through sexual body contact and given the protection against cervical cancer as the major objective of HPV immunization in adolescents, the factors children/women and sexuality, and subsequently reproduction and future generations were obviously present in the case of HPV vaccines from the onset. The initial immunization strategy focusing exclusively on girls further reinforced the social amplification of risk perception.[55] The media in some countries also portrayed the vaccine as "experimental".[56] Novelty, uncertainty and scientific debate are further cognitive factors increasing risk perception.[57] On the whole, the presence of cognitive factors for HPV vaccines was predictive of the need for a specific and careful communication strategy.

In the scientific as well as general media concerns were raised indeed over benefit, i.e. vaccine effectiveness long-term, effects on natural immunity, future HPV strain replacement,[58, 59, 60, 61, 62, 63] as well as over safety.[64] Safety concerns discussed in many different countries related

---

[54] Bennett P. Understanding responses to risk: some basic findings. In: Bennett P, Calman K. Risk communication and public health. Oxford: Oxford University Press; 1999. (Quoting Fischhhoff B, Slovic P, Lichtenstein S, Read S, Coombes B. How safe is safe enough?: a psychometric study of attitudes towards technological risks and benefits. Policy Science. 1978,9: 127-152.; Gardner GT, Gould LC. Public perceptions of risks and benefits of technology. Risk Analysis. 1989, 9: 225-242.; Slovic P. Informing and educating about risks. Risk Analysis. 1986; 6: 403-415.)

[55] Thompson M. Who's guarding what? – a post-structural feminist analysis of Gardasil discourses. Health Commun. 2010, 25: 119-130.

[56] Rondy M, van Lier A, van de Kassteele J, Rust L, de Melker H. Determinants for HPV vaccine uptake in the Netherlands: A multilevel study. Vaccine. 2010,28: 2070-2075.

[57] Bennett P. Understanding responses to risk: some basic findings. In: Bennett P, Calman K. Risk communication and public health. Oxford: Oxford University Press; 1999. (Quoting Fischhhoff B, Slovic P, Lichtenstein S, Read S, Coombes B. How safe is safe enough?: a psychometric study of attitudes towards technological risks and benefits. Policy Science. 1978, 9: 127-152.; Gardner GT, Gould LC. Public perceptions of risks and benefits of technology. Risk Analysis. 1989, 9: 225-242.; Slovic P. Informing and educating about risks. Risk Analysis. 1986; 6: 403-415.)

[58] Rondy M, van Lier A, van de Kassteele J, Rust L, de Melker H. Determinants for HPV vaccine uptake in the Netherlands: A multilevel study. Vaccine. 2010, 28: 2070-2075.

[59] Gerhardus A, Razum O. A long story made too short: surrogate variables and the communication of HPV vaccine trial results. J Epidemiol Community Health. 2010, 64: 377-378.

[60] Nghi NQ, Lamontagne DS, Bingham A, Rafiq M, Mai le TP, Lien NT, Khanh NC, Hong DT, Huyen DT, Tho NT, Hien NT. Human papillomavirus vaccine introduction in Vietnam: formative research findings. Sex Health. 2010, 7: 262-270.

[61] Rothman SM, Rothman DJ. Marketing HPV vaccine: implications for adolescent health and medical professionalism. J Am Med Assoc. 2009, 302: 781-786.

[62] Sherris J, Friedman A, Wittet S, Davies P, Steben M, Saraiya M. Education, training, and communication for HPV vaccines. Vaccine. 2006, 24 Suppl 3: S3 210-218 (chapter 25).

[63] Tafuri S, Martinelli D, Vece MM, Quarto M, Germinario C, Prato R. Communication skills in HPV prevention: an audit among Italian healthcare workers. Vaccine. 2010, 28: 5609-5613.

[64] Friedman AL, Shepeard H. Exploring the knowledge, attitudes, beliefs, and communication preferences of the general public regarding HPV: findings from CDC focus group research and implications for practice. Health Educ Behav. 2007, 34: 471-485.

to the exposure of "young girls",[65] to the burden of "too many vaccines",[66] and to the potential for adverse reactions,[67, 68, 69, 70] fatal outcomes[71] and long-term safety.[72] A specific concern was voiced about the impact of the vaccine on female fertility.[73] In low resource healthcare settings concerns over vaccine product quality, use of expired products and unsafe injection added to the fears.[74] Beyond quality and safety, social concerns arose that HPV immunization would increase early and multi-partner sexual activity.[75, 76, 77]

In any case, communicating about HPV immunization requires addressing intimate matters with young people, including whether sexual activity has started or not, and this constitutes a communication challenge in and of itself.[78] Some of the initial public concerns could in the meantime be addressed by evidence from long-term and real-life research in the period after licensure and launch of the HPV vaccines.[79] Also an increase of unsafe sexual activity or negative pregnancy outcomes could be refuted.[80, 81]

One might wonder if despite all the awareness one had or could have had with looking at the HPV vaccine launch from a cognitive factors perspective, whether communication strategies at launch were optimal in all countries and in particular whether they supported adequately healthcare professionals (HCPs). HCPs might have felt pretty alone with all the questions raised in the public domain, having to talk to young people about intimate matters and overcoming vaccine anxiety of individuals arising from both these constellations. HCPs need most certainly to be provided with in-depth information from the vaccine development phase onwards, as they often prefer to form their own conclusions. Nowadays researches get increasingly involved in surveys prior to HPV vaccination programs to inform the information campaigns.[82]

---

[65] Tafuri S, Martinelli D, Vece MM, Quarto M, Germinario C, Prato R. Communication skills in HPV prevention: an audit among Italian healthcare workers. Vaccine. 2010, 28: 5609-5613.

[66] Sherris J, Friedman A, Wittet S, Davies P, Steben M, Saraiya M. Education, training, and communication for HPV vaccines. Vaccine. 2006, 24 Suppl 3: S3 210-218 (chapter 25).

[67] Bingham A, Drake JK, LaMontagne DS. Sociocultural issues in the introduction of human papillomavirus vaccine in low-resource settings. Arch Pediatr Adolesc Med. 2009, 163: 455-461.

[68] Brown EC, Little P, Leydon GM. Communication challenges of HPV vaccination. Fam Pract. 2010, 27: 224-229.

[69] Chow SN, Soon R, Park JS, Pancharoen C, Qiao YL, Basu P, Ngan HY. Knowledge, attitudes, and communication around human papillomavirus (HPV) vaccination amongst urban Asian mothers and physicians. Vaccine. 2010, 28: 3809-3817.

[70] Rondy M, van Lier A, van de Kassteele J, Rust L, de Melker H. Determinants for HPV vaccine uptake in the Netherlands: A multilevel study. Vaccine. 2010, 28: 2070-2075.

[71] Nghi NQ, Lamontagne DS, Bingham A, Rafiq M, Mai le TP, Lien NT, Khanh NC, Hong DT, Huyen DT, Tho NT, Hien NT. Human papillomavirus vaccine introduction in Vietnam: formative research findings. Sex Health. 2010, 7: 262-270.

[72] Brown EC, Little P, Leydon GM. Communication challenges of HPV vaccination. Fam Pract. 2010, 27: 224-229.

[73] Nghi NQ, Lamontagne DS, Bingham A, Rafiq M, Mai le TP, Lien NT, Khanh NC, Hong DT, Huyen DT, Tho NT, Hien NT. Human papillomavirus vaccine introduction in Vietnam: formative research findings. Sex Health. 2010, 7: 262-270.

[74] Bingham A, Drake JK, LaMontagne DS. Sociocultural issues in the introduction of human papillomavirus vaccine in low-resource settings. Arch Pediatr Adolesc Med. 2009, 163: 455-461.

[75] Friedman AL, Shepeard H. Exploring the knowledge, attitudes, beliefs, and communication preferences of the general public regarding HPV: findings from CDC focus group research and implications for practice. Health Educ Behav. 2007, 34: 471-485.

[76] Sherris J, Friedman A, Wittet S, Davies P, Steben M, Saraiya M. Education, training, and communication for HPV vaccines. Vaccine. 2006, 24 Suppl 3: S3 210-218 (chapter 25).

[77] Tafuri S, Martinelli D, Vece MM, Quarto M, Germinario C, Prato R. Communication skills in HPV prevention: an audit among Italian healthcare workers. Vaccine. 2010, 28: 5609-5613.

[78] Brown EC, Little P, Leydon GM. Communication challenges of HPV vaccination. Fam Pract. 2010, 27: 224-229.

[79] World Health Organization (WHO). Global Advisory Committee on Vaccine Safety Statement on safety of HPV vaccines. Genève: WHO, 17 December 2015. Accessible under: http://www.who.int/vaccine_safety/committee/topics/hpv/en/.

[80] Vázquez-Otero C. Dispelling the myth: exploring associations between the HPV vaccine and inconsistent condom use among college students. Prev Med. 2016, 93: 157-150.

[81] Hansen BT. No evidence that HPV vaccination leads to sexual risk compensation. Hum Vaccin Immunother. 2016, 12: 1451-1453.

[82] Example provided by Priya Bahri, European Medicines Agency (EMA).

CHAPTER 3.

PRODUCT LIFE-CYCLE MANAGEMENT APPROACH TO VACCINE SAFETY AND COMMUNICATION

3.1. Communication as part of vaccine pharmacovigilance

Vaccine pharmacovigilance has been defined as the science and activities relating to the detection, assessment, understanding and communication of adverse events following immunization and other vaccine- or immunization-related issues, and to the prevention of untoward effects of the vaccine or immunization.[83] Communication about potential risks, demonstrated safety and measures to minimize risks, and programmes to support safe and effective use of vaccines, here referred to as "vaccine safety communication," are therefore a recognized part of pharmacovigilance. So far, for all medicinal products, the implementation of established principles and guidance on communication processes has been slow and incomplete worldwide.[84, 85]

Fundamental to achieving the aims of vaccine safety communication (see §2.1) is addressing not only safety concerns identified by specialists, but also those concerns voiced by the general public, (potential) vaccinees and their parents as well as healthcare professional (HCP). A strategic approach to vaccine safety communication with collaborative links between all stakeholders has been proposed for medicinal products in general[86] and for vaccines in particular[87] (see Chapter 4). This can be integrated with the processes for monitoring and assessing the benefit-risk balances of vaccines, so that concerns and information needs voiced by the public are included in benefit-risk monitoring and assessments.

Data to be communicated are not only those about safety itself but also those contextualizing a risk or an AEFI case(s), e.g. with data on disease epidemiology, vaccine use/exposure rates, baseline rates of events which can occur with and without vaccination and baseline pregnancy outcome data. A pharmacovigilance system therefore needs to collect such data not only for appropriate risk assessment, but also for communication. These data should be collected routinely and proactively, in order to allow for quick and valid assessments (see Example 2.3).

For effective communication and trust-building, it is likewise fundamental to be transparent in relation to the public about the pharmacovigilance processes in place, the available data, remaining uncertainties

---

[83] Council for International Organizations of Medical Sciences (CIOMS). Definition and application of terms of vaccine pharmacovigilance (report of CIOMS/WHO Working Group on Vaccine Pharmacovigilance). Geneva: CIOMS, 2012. Accessible at: https://cioms.ch/shop/product/definitions-and-applications-of-terms-for-vaccine-pharmacovigilance/

[84] Bahri P, Harrison-Woolrych M. Focussing on risk communication about medicines [editorial]. Drug Saf. 2012, 35: 971-975.

[85] Bahri P, Dodoo AN, Edwards BD, Edwards IR, Fermont I, Hagemann U, Hartigan-Go K, Hugman B, Mol PG (on behalf of the ISoP CommSIG). The ISoP CommSIG for improving medicinal product risk communication: a new special interest group of the International Society of Pharmacovigilance. Drug Saf. 2015, 38: 621-627.

[86] Bahri P. Public pharmacovigilance communication: a process calling for evidence-based, objective-driven strategies. Drug Saf. 2010, 33: 1065-1079.

[87] Larson H. The globalization of risk and risk perception: why we need a new model of risk communication for vaccines. Drug Saf. 2012, 35: 1053-1059.

and the rationale for decisions taken. It must be demonstrated that the pharmacovigilance processes and data are robust and conducted in an unbiased manner (see Example 4.3.2 concerning the HPV vaccine media monitoring at EMA).

Vaccine safety communication is a task that is continuously necessary during the entire life-cycle of a vaccine product, beginning at the time of vaccine development, especially crucial at the time of licensure/launch and to be maintained long-term throughout the post-licensure phase. As the safety data base for a vaccine will increase over time, but also new safety concerns may be identified, the messages to be communicated will evolve throughout the life-cycle. Pharmacovigilance nowadays is increasingly proactive in collecting safety data and risk minimization through applying a risk management approach, for which planning should start already before a vaccine gets licensed for use (see §3.2).

3.2. Pre-licensure and launch phase

Two distinct processes occur when a new vaccine first becomes publicly available. One is the licensure[88] by relevant regulatory authorities to ensure that a product is of ensured quality, safety and efficacy and to specify the conditions for its safe and effective launch and usage in this jurisdiction in public and private healthcare. The second is the launch of the vaccine by immunization programs in wide or focused target populations in order to achieve specified diseases control and health objectives. Sometimes, in countries of limited regulatory resources and/or other regulatory priorities, vaccines will be launched in immunization programs relying on prior licensure in well-established jurisdictions, without separate local licensure.[89]

Public awareness about a vaccine product may already begin prior to licensure and launch in early clinical development of a vaccine, particularly if it is being developed in response to an unmet health need or a current public health emergency. Examples are the malaria vaccine and the Ebola vaccines. The development of the latter has been catalysed by the West African Ebola epidemic of 2014/2015, and overall results from both phase 1 and 2 studies were communicated by various media outlets, although no single vaccine had yet been authorized (see Example 3.2.1).

Example 3.2.1: The need for understanding concerns in different communities over the Ebola virus and vaccines prior to launching clinical trials

> In response to the Ebola virus outbreak in West Africa in 2014, several candidate vaccines that had demonstrated efficacy in animal models and could be produced at clinical grade, were evaluated through a series of clinical trials. From the third quarter of 2014, phase 1 trials were conducted concurrently in North America and Europe as well as in some African countries that were not affected by the outbreak. By the first quarter of 2015, three phase 3 trials were

---

[88] The terms "approval", "authorization" and "licensure" in the context of vaccine (and drug) regulation in different jurisdictions mean the declaration by a regulatory authority that a product following review was found to have a positive benefit-risk profile and is approved for marketing and use. For consistency we have adopted "licensure" to cover any of these regulatory procedures or declarations. "Marketing" (or "post-marketing", etc.) is usually used to describe the phase of vaccine distribution following the manufacturer's decision to market the vaccine. The manufacturer may decide not to market a product even though licensure has been granted by the regulatory authority. While "marketing" differs in meaning, we have adopted, for consistency, the terms "pre-licensure" and "post-licensure" throughout this report to include everything that follows licensing of the product (i.e. "post-licensure" includes post-marketing considerations that would apply in the specific context in which the term is used) (see Council for International Organizations of Medical Sciences (CIOMS). Definition and application of terms of vaccine pharmacovigilance (report of CIOMS/WHO Working Group on Vaccine Pharmacovigilance). Geneva: CIOMS, 2012. Accessible at: https://cioms.ch/shop/product/definitions-and-applications-of-terms-for-vaccine-pharmacovigilance/.

[89] Council for International Organizations of Medical Sciences (CIOMS). CIOMS Guide to Active Vaccine Safety Surveillance (report of the CIOMS Working Group on Vaccine Safety). Geneva: CIOMS, 2017, Appendix I: Essential Vaccine Information, pp.57-59.

Guidance Summary 3.2.2: Types of risk minimization measures for medicinal products

Product information:

- Package leaflet
- Product information for healthcare professionals (e.g. in the EU this is the summary of product characteristics (SmPC))[95]
- Labelling on the outer packaging
- Pack size and design
- Educational materials
- Direct healthcare professional communications (DHPC)[96]
- Legal status of the product, e.g. prescription-only
- Controlled access programs

The application of risk minimization measures to vaccines can be more challenging. For example the leaflet for the patient is rarely handed over to the vaccinee or the carer as part of the package, because, unlike for other medicinal products, vaccines are often not provided to individuals in the pharmacy but administered immediately in the clinic or another vaccination site. An example is provided of a risk management plan for a vaccine assessed in the European Union (EU) in collaboration with WHO in Example 3.2.2. Consideration has to be given as to how to communicate the safety advice in the package leaflet amongst carers, to ensure that any possible risks are avoided and that carers know how to limit the impact of an adverse reaction should it occur. This may be an objective of a Vaccine Safety Communication Plan (see Chapter 4).

Example 3.2.2: Risk management planning for DTPw-HBV quadrivalent vaccine

A quadrivalent combined bacterial and viral vaccine protecting against diphtheria, tetanus, pertussis and hepatitis B, and was assessed by the European Medicines Agency (EMA) in collaboration with WHO, in order to facilitate its use in countries outside the European Union (EU). Based on the clinical trials, the following was classified as 'important identified risks': allergic reactions, high fever, convulsions, hypotonic-hyporesponsive episodes; and the following as 'important potential risks': apnoea in prematurely born children, fainting, brain disorder. In addition, the lack of safety and immunogenicity in children born prematurely was classified as 'missing information'. Given these safety specifications, no risk minimization measures other than the product information were considered necessary.[97] Information on the identified and potential risks, including warnings and precautions for use to minimize their occurrence and

---

[95] European Medicines Agency (EMA) and Heads of Medicines Agencies. Guideline on good pharmacovigilance practices - Module XVI, Rev 2: Risk minimisation measures: selection of tools and effectiveness indicators. London: EMA, 2017. Accessible at: http://www.ema.europa.eu/ema/index.jsp?curl=pages/regulation/document_listing/document_listing_000345.jsp&mid=WC0b01ac058058f32c.

[96] DHPC is considered an additional risk minimization measure beyond routine measures. For more information, see CIOMS IX Report on Risk Minimisation for Medicinal Products, Geneva, Switzerland, 2014.

[97] European Medicines Agency (EMA). Summary of the risk management plan (RMP) for Tritanrix HB [Diphtheria, tetanus, pertussis (whole cell) and hepatitis B (rDNA) vaccine (adsorbed)]. London: EMA, 2014. Accessible at: http://www.ema.europa.eu/docs/en_GB/document_library/Medicine_for_use_outside_EU/2014/03/WC500163201.pdf.

and the rationale for decisions taken. It must be demonstrated that the pharmacovigilance processes and data are robust and conducted in an unbiased manner (see Example 4.3.2 concerning the HPV vaccine media monitoring at EMA).

Vaccine safety communication is a task that is continuously necessary during the entire life-cycle of a vaccine product, beginning at the time of vaccine development, especially crucial at the time of licensure/launch and to be maintained long-term throughout the post-licensure phase. As the safety data base for a vaccine will increase over time, but also new safety concerns may be identified, the messages to be communicated will evolve throughout the life-cycle. Pharmacovigilance nowadays is increasingly proactive in collecting safety data and risk minimization through applying a risk management approach, for which planning should start already before a vaccine gets licensed for use (see §3.2).

3.2. Pre-licensure and launch phase

Two distinct processes occur when a new vaccine first becomes publicly available. One is the licensure[88] by relevant regulatory authorities to ensure that a product is of ensured quality, safety and efficacy and to specify the conditions for its safe and effective launch and usage in this jurisdiction in public and private healthcare. The second is the launch of the vaccine by immunization programs in wide or focused target populations in order to achieve specified diseases control and health objectives. Sometimes, in countries of limited regulatory resources and/or other regulatory priorities, vaccines will be launched in immunization programs relying on prior licensure in well-established jurisdictions, without separate local licensure.[89]

Public awareness about a vaccine product may already begin prior to licensure and launch in early clinical development of a vaccine, particularly if it is being developed in response to an unmet health need or a current public health emergency. Examples are the malaria vaccine and the Ebola vaccines. The development of the latter has been catalysed by the West African Ebola epidemic of 2014/2015, and overall results from both phase 1 and 2 studies were communicated by various media outlets, although no single vaccine had yet been authorized (see Example 3.2.1).

Example 3.2.1: The need for understanding concerns in different communities over the Ebola virus and vaccines prior to launching clinical trials

> In response to the Ebola virus outbreak in West Africa in 2014, several candidate vaccines that had demonstrated efficacy in animal models and could be produced at clinical grade, were evaluated through a series of clinical trials. From the third quarter of 2014, phase 1 trials were conducted concurrently in North America and Europe as well as in some African countries that were not affected by the outbreak. By the first quarter of 2015, three phase 3 trials were

---

[88] The terms "approval", "authorization" and "licensure" in the context of vaccine (and drug) regulation in different jurisdictions mean the declaration by a regulatory authority that a product following review was found to have a positive benefit-risk profile and is approved for marketing and use. For consistency we have adopted "licensure" to cover any of these regulatory procedures or declarations. "Marketing" (or "post-marketing", etc.) is usually used to describe the phase of vaccine distribution following the manufacturer's decision to market the vaccine. The manufacturer may decide not to market a product even though licensure has been granted by the regulatory authority. While "marketing" differs in meaning, we have adopted, for consistency, the terms "pre-licensure" and "post-licensure" throughout this report to include everything that follows licensing of the product (i.e. "post-licensure" includes post-marketing considerations that would apply in the specific context in which the term is used) (see Council for International Organizations of Medical Sciences (CIOMS). Definition and application of terms of vaccine pharmacovigilance (report of CIOMS/WHO Working Group on Vaccine Pharmacovigilance). Geneva: CIOMS, 2012. Accessible at: https://cioms.ch/shop/product/definitions-and-applications-of-terms-for-vaccine-pharmacovigilance/.

[89] Council for International Organizations of Medical Sciences (CIOMS). CIOMS Guide to Active Vaccine Safety Surveillance (report of the CIOMS Working Group on Vaccine Safety). Geneva: CIOMS, 2017, Appendix I: Essential Vaccine Information, pp.57-59.

initiated in the three most affected countries (Liberia, Sierra Leone and Guinea). Despite the unprecedented pace in a vaccine clinical development process, these trials complied with good clinical practices that are today expected in clinical research.

Planning and implementing those vaccine efficacy trials involved several communication challenges related to what was known about the vaccines, the selection of vaccine recipients and controls, and respecting an informed consent of participants with limited literacy. The general acceptability of the intervention was also subject to concern initially, as outbreak control measures had been complicated by traditional rituals, perception of disease transmission and mistrust on the part of several communities.

In each country, investigation teams, including communication professionals, worked closely with political and religious leaders to identify perception issues related to prevention of Ebola virus disease and use of an experimental vaccine, serving as advocates for the population. Local workers and communities were engaged to present the study purposes. Where the protocol included vaccination of frontline workers, national and local public figures were vaccinated early in some trials to ease population concerns and to indicate that supporting the evaluation of vaccines against Ebola virus was a collective responsibility[90].

At the time of licensure, knowledge about the safety of a vaccine is still limited. Most vaccine trials are designed with a primary objective for efficacy, and their typical size of a couple of thousands subjects limits the detection of adverse events to those that occur at a frequency $> 1/1000$.[91] As a result, most of the safety information included in the product label is limited to those events that occur in $1/10$ - $1/100$ patients, and largely these events describe the expected local injection site reactions and systemic events of fever and malaise.

In contrast, post-licensure use of vaccines is widespread with exposure in up to millions of subjects. Therefore, even adverse events occurring more rarely, between $1/1,000$ - $1/10,000$, and thus not observed in clinical trials, may affect thousands of individuals. Furthermore, most pre-licensure clinical trials exclude certain populations, such as premature infants, pregnant women, or people with underlying medical conditions. However, after launch vaccines are usually given universally and may be, depending on the vaccine type and disease to prevent, encouraged in precisely those populations excluded from clinical trials, e.g. pregnant women or older patients with multiple diseases.

Therefore it is crucial, prior to licensure, to adequately explore and document the gaps in the safety database and plan how to fill these as quickly as possible in the post-licensure phase. Also it needs to be planned how to minimize and prevent harm from identified or potential risks. A risk management approach supports documenting how data are collected and risk minimization measures are implemented and to decide, in the light of the results, if and how vaccine safety needs to be further improved. While requirements for risk management systems may be tailored to the specific needs and environment of a country, the concept is universal (see Guidance Summary 3.2.1). There a number of risk minimization measures available for medicines (see Guidance Summary 3.2.2), and they mostly require communication for their implementation.

---

[90] Example provided by Dr. Andrea Vicari, Advisor Epidemic-Prone Diseases, Pan American Health Organization (formerly at WHO HQ), per communication with Dr. Patrick Zuber, 28/08/2017.

[91] European Medicines Agency (EMA). CHMP note for guidance on the clinical evaluation of vaccines. London: EMA, 2005.

Guidance Summary 3.2.1: Concept of risk management systems for medicinal products

A major conceptual example for risk management systems comes from the European Union (EU). An EU risk management system was defined for the pharmaceutical sector first in 2005 and later in legislation as a set of pharmacovigilance activities and interventions designed to identify, characterize, prevent or minimize risks relating to a medicinal product, including the assessment of the effectiveness of those interventions[92] (see Figure 3.2).

The submission of risk management plans describing product-specific risk management systems have become a regulatory requirement for applicants/ marketing authorization holders in the EU, commonly known as EU-RMP. These have to be submitted, using a defined template, with the licensure application for every new medicinal product (including new generics) or for existing products with a major safety concern. An EU-RMP describes what is known and not known about the safety profile of the concerned medicinal product, indicates how so-called missing information will be filled and the safety profile of the product further characterized through future data collection, and demands measures to be taken for prevention or minimizing identified or potential risks (see Guidance Summary 3.2.2). Summaries of the risk management plans for the public are made available on the European Medicine Agency's website.[93]

Figure 3.2: Risk management cycle

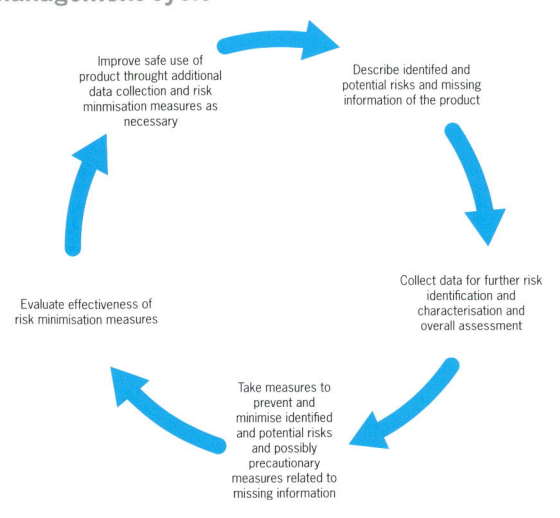

- Describe identifed and potential risks and missing information of the product
- Collect data for further risk identification and characterisation and overall assessment
- Take measures to prevent and minimise identified and potential risks and possibly precautionary measures related to missing information
- Evaluate effectiveness of risk minimisation measures
- Improve safe use of product throught additional data collection and risk minmisation measures as necessary

Source: European Medicines Agency, 2012.[94]

---

[92] Directive 2001/83/EC of the European Parliament and of the Council, Article 1(28b).

[93] European Medicines Agency and Heads of Medicines Agencies. Guideline on good pharmacovigilance practices - Module V Revision 2: Risk management systems. Accessible at: http://www.ema.europa.eu/ema/index.jsp?curl=pages/regulation/document_listing/document_listing_000345.jsp&mid=WC0b01ac058058f32c.

[94] European Medicines Agency (EMA) and Heads of Medicines Agencies. Guideline on good pharmacovigilance practices - Module V: Risk management systems. EMA/838713/2011. London: EMA, 2012. 20 February 2012, p.7. Accessible at: http://www.ema.europa.eu/docs/en_GB/document_library/Scientific_guideline/2012/02/WC500123208.pdf.

Guidance Summary 3.2.2: Types of risk minimization measures for medicinal products

Product information:

- Package leaflet
- Product information for healthcare professionals (e.g. in the EU this is the summary of product characteristics (SmPC))[95]
- Labelling on the outer packaging
- Pack size and design
- Educational materials
- Direct healthcare professional communications (DHPC)[96]
- Legal status of the product, e.g. prescription-only
- Controlled access programs

The application of risk minimization measures to vaccines can be more challenging. For example the leaflet for the patient is rarely handed over to the vaccinee or the carer as part of the package, because, unlike for other medicinal products, vaccines are often not provided to individuals in the pharmacy but administered immediately in the clinic or another vaccination site. An example is provided of a risk management plan for a vaccine assessed in the European Union (EU) in collaboration with WHO in Example 3.2.2. Consideration has to be given as to how to communicate the safety advice in the package leaflet amongst carers, to ensure that any possible risks are avoided and that carers know how to limit the impact of an adverse reaction should it occur. This may be an objective of a Vaccine Safety Communication Plan (see Chapter 4).

Example 3.2.2: Risk management planning for DTPw-HBV quadrivalent vaccine

A quadrivalent combined bacterial and viral vaccine protecting against diphtheria, tetanus, pertussis and hepatitis B, and was assessed by the European Medicines Agency (EMA) in collaboration with WHO, in order to facilitate its use in countries outside the European Union (EU). Based on the clinical trials, the following was classified as 'important identified risks': allergic reactions, high fever, convulsions, hypotonic-hyporesponsive episodes; and the following as 'important potential risks': apnoea in prematurely born children, fainting, brain disorder. In addition, the lack of safety and immunogenicity in children born prematurely was classified as 'missing information'. Given these safety specifications, no risk minimization measures other than the product information were considered necessary.[97] Information on the identified and potential risks, including warnings and precautions for use to minimize their occurrence and

---

[95] European Medicines Agency (EMA) and Heads of Medicines Agencies. Guideline on good pharmacovigilance practices - Module XVI, Rev 2: Risk minimisation measures: selection of tools and effectiveness indicators. London: EMA, 2017. Accessible at: http://www.ema.europa.eu/ema/index.jsp?curl=pages/regulation/document_listing/document_listing_000345.jsp&mid=WC0b01ac058058f32c.

[96] DHPC is considered an additional risk minimization measure beyond routine measures. For more information, see CIOMS IX Report on Risk Minimisation for Medicinal Products, Geneva, Switzerland, 2014.

[97] European Medicines Agency (EMA). Summary of the risk management plan (RMP) for Tritanrix HB [Diphtheria, tetanus, pertussis (whole cell) and hepatitis B (rDNA) vaccine (adsorbed)]. London: EMA, 2014. Accessible at: http://www.ema.europa.eu/docs/en_GB/document_library/Medicine_for_use_outside_EU/2014/03/WC500163201.pdf.

severity of impact, has been included in the package leaflets for carers and the healthcare professional information.[98, 99]

The next example (Example 3.2.3) demonstrates a successful launch of a new vaccine in India in a climate of controversy in the public domain. While the example is taken from an immunization program rather than communication by a regulatory authority, the approach taken to work with stakeholders is equally applicable to pharmacovigilance.

Example 3.2.3: The introduction of pentavalent vaccines in Kerala, India, supported by close interactions with the healthcare community and the media

Pentavalent vaccines, protecting against five potentially deadly diseases, namely diphtheria, tetanus, pertussis, hepatitis B and *Haemophilus influenzae* type b (Hib), have been introduced successfully in India. Some federal states became even early adopters with the help of communication efforts, despite controversies prior to launch. Some individuals, active in alternative medicine but also other healthcare professionals, questioned the utility and safety of the vaccines, and mainstream daily newspapers joined in, opposing the introduction of the vaccines in the State of Kerala.

In response, a committee of local paediatricians and community doctors was constituted, to examine in detail the issues raised and to prepare a full assessment of the benefit-risk balance of pentavalent vaccines, taking into account the burden of infectious diseases and all available published and unpublished data on the vaccines. The committee concluded that the benefit-risk balance was positive, and a comprehensive communication strategy was applied.

This strategy started with a workshop, convened by the State and with support of UNICEF, on 17 November 2011, with the officers from State departments, the heads of the paediatric and community medicine of all medical colleagues and further concerned officials, to present the report. Immunization guidelines, comprehensively addressing not only information on the vaccine products themselves, but also on safe injection technique, cold chain requirements and surveillance of potential adverse events, were disseminated in English and the local language. Immunization cards with the correct dosing were disseminated as well.

This was accompanied by actual assessment of the equipment, a wide-reaching training programme and a supervision plan for the daily monitoring of the immunization programme. Further advocacy workshops were organized and a number of mass communication materials in print and electronically were disseminated: posters, booklets and displays in major daily newspapers. In areas of known vaccine hesitancy, closer interactions with these communities were sought at various levels, including with those active in media folk arts and healthcare.

As regards interacting with the media, a specific press-conference was held to present the committee report, and the fact that this was called by the Minister of Health demonstrated highest leadership and commitment to safe immunization. This was followed up by media sensitization activities prior to launch of the immunization programme, and these helped to reduce undue criticism over vaccine safety in the media. Even when later, one baby sadly died post-vaccination (note: death proved to be unrelated), the media reported on the examinations done and the fact that all other children who had been vaccinated from the same vial were healthy, and continued engaging in immunization advocacy.

---

[98] European Medicines Agency (EMA). Trintanrix HB: product information. London: EMA, 2014. Accessible at: http://www.ema.europa.eu/docs/en_GB/document_library/Medicine_for_use_outside_EU/2014/03/WC500163198.pdf.

[99] Example provided by Priya Bahri, European Medicines Agency, London, United Kingdom.

However, a communication strategy is never completed. As pharmacovigilance is a continuous activity in the post-authorization phase of vaccines as of all other medicines, so is communication with the public.

The events in the media in India after the successful launch of the immunization programme in Kerala in 2012 illustrate this. Routine media monitoring revealed the following: of the 383 news stories on the pentavalent vaccine in all India from January 2013 onward, 57% coverage was positive, while 21.5% coverage negative. In the course of 2013 however an increased tendency of the media to hold the vaccine responsible for deaths and to portray the vaccine sensationally was observed. Overall in 2013, 40% of the media coverage was negative.

A consistent lack of correct reporting on the vaccine and a need of re-sensitizing the media about the importance of immunization was identified. As a result, UNICEF along with its partners, held a series of media sensitization workshops and roundtable discussions in major cities across India, i.e. in New Delhi, Chandigarh, Lucknow, Chennai, Raipur, Patna, Bhopal, Jaipur, Kolkata and Guwahati. A number of senior editors from the print, electronic and broadcast media operating in Hindi or English were engaged. Guidance for spokespersons about how to interact with the media during an investigation of an adverse event following immunization was also provided at trainings for immunization officers. A number of field visits of senior journalists were organized to various states and hard to reach area in Assam, Jharkhand, Uttar Pradesh, Bihar, Odisha and Madhya Pradesh, among others.

An analysis of print media articles conducted after this engagement with the media on routine immunization issues revealed that, compared to 2013, positive coverage on the pentavalent vaccine increased in 2014 by 126% and the negative coverage on the vaccine fell by 66%. This was also partly due to the parallel media engagement being undertaken for "Mission Indradhanush," the Indian government's initiative launched in December 2014 to ensure that all children under the age of two and pregnant women are fully immunised with all available vaccines.[100] There was an increase in balanced coverage and the tendency of the media to hold pentavalent vaccine responsible for deaths also fell. While the vaccine was held responsible for AEFIs in 58% of media-reported cases in 2013, the media pointed at pentavalent vaccines as responsible in only 31% in 2014. The media analysis findings corroborate the effectiveness of sensitizing the media.[101]

3.3. Post-licensure phase

While at the time of licensure there is enough evidence to conclude a positive risk-benefit balance, uncertainty regarding some aspects of the risks remain (see §3.2). When a product is launched, there is however often little communication to the public about the knowledge gaps. Communications typically address the identified and sometimes potential risks, which were observed in clinical trials and have been included in package labels, but communication regarding more theoretical potential risks and missing information in the safety database is usually lacking. With a view to transparency, it has been established that messages to the public should honestly acknowledge uncertainties and that it is better to do this proactively, rather than waiting for a debate in the scientific media to spill over into the general media.

During the post-licensure phase, the knowledge gaps get filled as safety data are obtained from both passive surveillance systems (i.e. spontaneous reporting) and active systems (i.e. active safety

---

[100] Mission Indradhanush: Centre asks all private TV, radio channels to promote government's immunisation programme The Financial Express PTI | New Delhi | Published: July 30, 2017. http://www.financialexpress.com/india-news/mission-indradhanush-centre-asks-all-private-tv-radio-channels-to-promote-governments-immunisation-programme/786539/.

[101] Example provided by Sonia Sarkar, UNICEF India.

surveillance and epidemiological post-authorization safety studies),[102] including those required by a risk management plan if applicable (see §3.2). Safety signals[103] identified from spontaneous reporting systems often require subsequent epidemiological studies to quantify or to further characterize the risk. However, most AEFIs detected from spontaneous reporting are so rare (i.e. 1/10,000 - 1/100,000) that follow-up epidemiological studies lack feasibility and statistical power or require significant cooperation for collecting data from multiple database sources. Nevertheless, often these types of rare events garner the majority of public attention in the media. Transparency and clear communication throughout the evaluation of post-licensure safety signals is essential for the maintenance of public trust in the vaccine safety processes and provide for informed choice.

With increasing post-licensure experience, knowledge of the safety profile of the vaccine increases, and uncertainty decreases. With an acceptable safety profile and a successful communication strategy, many vaccines receive general public acceptance in the long run. However, safety signals may continue to arise which can for example be attributable to quality issues in the manufacturing process, the introduction of new vaccines used in combination with older vaccines, or the expansion of a vaccine indication to new populations. Communication strategies must be adaptable to new needs; simply repeating a previous, general message (i.e. "this vaccine is safe") is not adequate to ensure continued public trust.

Examples for how communication has been handled successfully in relation to vaccine safety concerns arising in the post-licensure phase are provided below (see Examples 3.3.1 and 3.3.2).

Example 3.3.1: Addressing the risk of febrile seizures with a serogroup B meningococcal vaccines in the United Kingdom

A vaccine against meningococcal serotype B was licensed by the European Medicines Agency (EMA) in 2013. Within the clinical trial program an increased rate of high fevers and febrile seizures in those infants who received this vaccine in combination with routine infant immunizations was noted. These risks were included in the package leaflet with a frequency of > 1/100 and < 1/1000. Additionally, risk minimization measures to prevent fever and subsequent seizures were described in the package leaflet as follows: "Your doctor or nurse may ask you to give your child medicines that lower fever at the time and after [the vaccine] has been given. This will help to reduce some of the side effects of [the vaccine]."

The UK was the primary country within the European Union which incorporated the meningococcal B vaccine into its routine childhood vaccination program, and in September 2015 infants started receiving the vaccination at 2 and 4 months of age in combination with pentavalent, pneumococcal, and rotavirus vaccines. Active measures were taken by Public Health England to inform both healthcare professionals and parents about the need for use of prophylactic paracetamol at the time of vaccination. Healthcare professionals were provided both a protocol document as well as access to an instructional video that simulated a conversation between provider and parents. Parents were provided an information sheet at the time of discharge after delivery of a new baby as well as a patient information leaflet offering advice on the use of paracetamol.

---

[102] Council for International Organizations of Medical Sciences (CIOMS). CIOMS Guide to Active Vaccine Safety Surveillance (report of the CIOMS Working Group on Vaccine Safety). Geneva: CIOMS, 2017.

[103] A signal is defined as information that arises from one or multiple sources (including observations and experiments), which suggests a new potentially causal association or a new aspect of a known association between an intervention and an event or set of related events, either adverse or beneficial, that is judged to be of sufficient likelihood to justify verificatory action (see Council for International Organizations of Medical Sciences (CIOMS). Practical aspects of signal detection in pharmacovigilance. Geneva: CIOMS, 2010.). In the context of safety, a signal refers to an adverse event.

Below is the information leaflet which is distributed to parents at the time of vaccination with the meningococcal B vaccine.[104, 105]

Using paracetamol

to prevent and treat fever after MenB vaccination

NHS

My baby has just had the MenB vaccine, what should I expect now?

Fever can be expected after any vaccination, but is more common when the MenB vaccine (Bexsero) is given with the other routine vaccines at two and four months. Without paracetamol, more than half of infants will develop a temperature after these vaccines. The fever tends to peak around six hours after vaccination and is nearly always gone completely within two days. The fever shows the baby's immune system is responding to the vaccine, although the level of fever will depend on each child and does not show how well the vaccine will protect your baby.

How can I reduce the risk of fever?

Giving paracetamol soon after vaccination – and not waiting for a fever to develop – will reduce the risk of your child having a fever. With paracetamol, fewer than one in five children will get a fever and nearly all of these are mild (below 39°C). The paracetamol will also reduce the chance of your baby being irritable or suffering discomfort (such as pain at the site of the injection).

Which paracetamol product should I use?

You should use oral **infant paracetamol suspension. This kind of paracetamol comes in liquid form for use in babies and young children. It has a strength of 120mg/5ml.**

If you have not already got some paracetamol suspension for infants at home, you should get some from your local pharmacy or supermarket so that you can give the first dose of paracetamol within an hour of the vaccination. There are various products to choose from (including bottles and sachets) but the type needed is infant paracetamol suspension 120mg/5ml.

*(Note: Junior paracetamol (six plus) is stronger than infant paracetamol (250mg/5ml) and **must not** be used in babies.)*

After which vaccinations should I give my baby paracetamol?

Paracetamol is advised for your baby following the MenB vaccinations. The MenB vaccine is usually given at your baby's first and third immunisation appointments at two months and four months of age.

Paracetamol is not routinely needed after the Men B booster vaccine given at 12 months of age. By this age the baby's risk of fever is the same as after other vaccines.

How much paracetamol should I give?

A total of three doses of 2.5ml (60mg) of paracetamol are recommended following MenB vaccination. You should give the first dose at the time of vaccination or as soon as possible afterwards. You should then give the second dose of paracetamol around four to six hours later and a third dose four to six hours after that (see table). The 2.5ml dose should be measured and given either using a syringe or with a 2.5ml spoon (this is usually the small end of the spoon that comes in the pack).

For very premature babies (born before 32 weeks gestation), paracetamol should be prescribed by your doctor according to the infant's weight at the time of vaccination. You should check with your doctor and follow the instructions on the prescription.

Dosage and timing of infant paracetamol suspension (120mg/5ml) for use after primary MenB vaccinations (usually at two and four months of age)

Age of baby	Up to 6 months (usually at 2 and 4 months)
Dose 1	One 2.5ml (60mg) dose as soon as possible after vaccination
Dose 2	One 2.5ml (60mg) dose 4-6 hours after first dose
Dose 3	One 2.5ml (60mg) dose 4-6 hours after second dose

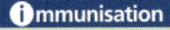

ⓘmmunisation

---

[104] Public Health England. MenB vaccine and paracetamol. Accessible at: https://www.gov.uk/government/publications/menb-vaccine-and-paracetamol.

[105] Example provided by Rebecca Chandler, Uppsala Monitoring Centre (UMC), Sweden, with confirmation by email 14 August 2017 to Karin Holm.

The advice in this leaflet only applies if your baby has had the MenB vaccine. If your baby has a fever at any other time you should follow the instructions and dose advice on the product packaging and patient information leaflet.

What if my baby still has a fever after having had the three doses of paracetamol?

Some babies may still develop fever after vaccination, even after having three doses of paracetamol. In the 48 hours after vaccination, if your baby still has a fever but is otherwise well, you can continue to give your baby the same 2.5 ml dose (60mg) of infant paracetamol (120mg/5ml) suspension.

- **You should always leave at least four hours between doses and never give more than four doses in any 24 hour period.**

You should also keep your baby cool by making sure they don't have too many layers of clothes or blankets, and give them lots of fluids. If your baby is breast-fed, the best fluid to give is breast milk.

- **If you are concerned about your baby's health at any time, then trust your instincts and speak to your GP or call NHS 111 in England and 0845 46 47 in Wales for advice.**
- **If your baby still has a fever more than 48 hours after vaccination you should speak to your GP or call NHS 111 in England and 0845 46 47 in Wales for advice.**

Other common questions:
Should I wake my baby to give paracetamol?

You should always try and give the first dose of paracetamol as soon as possible after the MenB vaccine. However if your baby is sleeping when the next doses are due, don't wake them up. You can give it when the baby next wakes as long as there is at least four hours between each dose.

Is it OK for small babies to have paracetamol?

Paracetamol is approved for managing fever in children from the age of two months. The patient information leaflet that comes with the pack may say that children aged two to three months should only be given two doses before talking to a doctor or pharmacist.

Although paracetamol is safe in very young children, the advice on the packaging is there to avoid parents giving paracetamol to a child with an unexplained fever. Such a fever could be a sign of a serious infection and treating this for too long may delay a parent seeking medical help.

As fever after vaccination is common, however, experts have advised that it is OK to give paracetamol for up to 48 hours after the MenB vaccine without seeking medical advice.

Fever in this time period is much more likely to be caused by the vaccine than by an infection. The paracetamol will also make your child feel better, and there is no risk of an over-dose provided you give no more than four 2.5ml doses in any 24 hour period.

Why does the manufacturer's patient information leaflet (PIL) contain different information?

You will find a patient information leaflet (PIL) in the supply of paracetamol you purchase. The PIL with the infant paracetamol suspension 120mg/5ml may provide different dosing instructions from the experts' recommendations for use following MenB vaccination. Here, in this leaflet, we give the details of the specific recommendations for the use of paracetamol following a MenB vaccination. For full information about the paracetamol product, please see the manufacturers PIL.

Does my baby need paracetamol with the booster vaccinations at 12 months?

By the age of 12 months your baby's risk of fever after MenB vaccine is the same as with the other vaccines. So, your baby does not need to take three doses of paracetamol with their routine 12 month vaccinations. However, if your baby does get fever at home or appears to be in discomfort, you can give your baby infant paracetamol using the dosing schedule for a child of that age as outlined on the instructions in the packet.

The advice to give more than two doses of paracetamol to babies aged two to three months only applies after the baby has had the MenB vaccine. If your baby has a fever at any other time, you should follow the instructions and dose advice on the product packaging and patient information leaflet.

NHS

© Crown copyright 2015

Example 3.3.2: Addressing the safety concern of narcolepsy for the H1N1 pandemic influenza vaccine used in Sweden

A number of cases of narcolepsy in children were observed during the early post-licensure phase of an H1N1 pandemic influenza vaccine used in late 2009. These cases were detected by passive surveillance systems in both Finland and Sweden, countries in which mass immunization practices had resulted in high vaccine uptake. Data for further characterisation and risk estimates were made available by active surveillance in the form of register-based studies designed in response to the initial signal, and the assessment outcome was communicated to the public.

A review of the lessons learned from the H1N1 pandemic influenza vaccine -narcolepsy experience was organized by the Swedish regulatory authority at a special symposium on narcolepsy research related to this vaccine in November 2014, which brought together multiple parties, including communication experts from the authority as well as representatives from the narcolepsy patient advocacy group.

Questions were asked of these representatives regarding the expected content, timing, process and channels for communication. In addition, they were asked about their impressions of the availability of experts at the authority to answer questions as well as how to best improve distribution of information to all parties in the future. Overall, the representatives felt that communication was of good quality but they would have liked clearer messages on the causal relationship rather than language including terms such as relative and absolute risks. There was also confusion regarding the roles of experts from different public bodies, like the regulatory authority and the public health authority. It was suggested that the regulatory authority should have corrected obviously misleading statements from opinion leaders in the public domain and the media through communication on its website as soon as possible.[106, 107]

---

[106] Feltelius N, Persson I, Ahlqvist-Rastad J, et al. A coordinated cross-disciplinary research initiative to address an increased incidence of narcolepsy following the 2009–2010 Pandemrix vaccination programme in Sweden. J Intern Med. 2015, 278: 335-353.

[107] Example provided by Rebecca Chandler, Uppsala Monitoring Centre (UMC), Sweden, personal communication by email 8 March 2016.

CHAPTER 4.
VACCINE SAFETY COMMUNICATION PLANS (VACSCPS)

4.1. Application of a strategic communication approach to vaccine safety

Strategic thinking has increasingly been applied worldwide to health communication since the 1980s. The process of strategic health communication can be divided in five steps, the P-Process of strategic health communication (Figure 4.1).

Figure 4.1: The P-Process of strategic health communication[108]

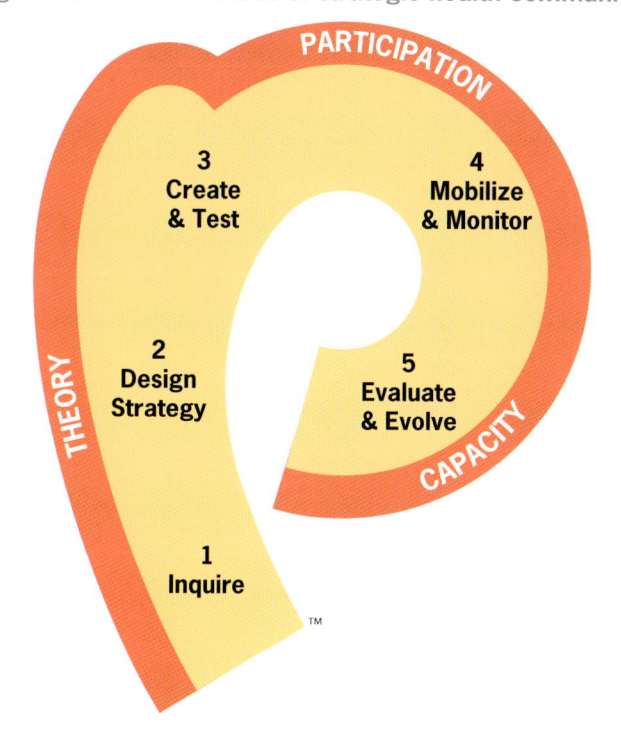

Step 1: Inquiry
- Analysis of the situation
- Management considerations

Step 2: Design strategy
- Agreement on communication objectives
- Communication plan

Step 3: Create & Test
- Communication materials

Step 4: Mobilize & Monitor
- Implementation of plan
- Dissemination of communication materials

Step 5: Evaluate & Evolve
- Evaluation if and how objectives have been achieved
- Evaluation of impact
- Updated communication plan

P stands for planning. It is essentially characterized by agreeing clear communication objectives as well as a communication plan designed to achieve these objectives, ideally in terms of desired behaviour.[109] A

---

[108] The Health Communication Capacity Collaborative. The P-Process: five steps to strategic communication. Baltimore, MD: Johns Hopkins Bloomberg School of Public Health Center for Communication Programs, 2013. Accessible at: http://www.thehealthcompass.org/sbcc-tools/p-process or http://ccp.jhu.edu/documents/P_Process_5_Steps.pdf.

[109] The Health Communication Capacity Collaborative. The P-Process: five steps to strategic communication. Baltimore: Johns Hopkins Bloomberg School of Public Health Center for Communication Programs, 2013. Accessible at: http://www.thehealthcompass.org/sbcc-tools/p-process.

call has been made to apply this approach to communication about safety of medicines in the regulatory environment,[110, 111, 112] as well as to public information for immunization programmes.[113] This strategic communication approach can also be used to create vaccine safety communication plans (VacSCP).

However, communication strategies are not generic 'one-size-fits-all', but require tailored messages and appropriate tools and channels to reach specific segments of the population, including hard-to-reach populations.[114] Research on vaccine hesitancy has also shown that sentiments are vaccine-type specific,[115] and political and social situations can change, as can the overall public health situation. For example, the situation where a continuation of successful vaccination is required for disease prevention, such as in the case of measles, differs from the situation of a public health emergency during a pandemic peak of a disease, and so the communication strategies will differ.

Different types of safety concerns will also require different responses, based on the evidence, which may call for precaution, risk minimization measures or disseminating reassuring information. Communication strategies for vaccines are more likely to succeed if they are integrated at local level with the provision of other community health needs.[116] Therefore the VacSCPs are to be designed specific to a vaccine-type and a given local situation at a specific point in time.

It might not be feasible for an organization to immediately develop and maintain VacSCPs for each vaccine, and a practical way is to create a generic plan suitable for the organization as a basis for generating vaccine-specific plans according to the given situation and priorities, e.g. according to current public health needs and the public debate. Key considerations for managers are listed in Checklist 4.1.

Checklist 4.1: Management considerations for VacSCPs

- ☑ Understand the situation and identify public health priorities
- ☑ Identify stakeholders including their roles and responsibilities
- ☑ Allocate budget
- ☑ Agree timeline for the implementation of the VacSCP
- ☑ Monitor the implementation of the VacSCP [117]

---

[110] Bahri P. Public pharmacovigilance communication: a process calling for evidence-based, objective-driven strategies. Drug Saf. 2010; 33: 1065-1079.

[111] Fischhoff B, Brewer NT, Downs JS. Communicating risks and benefits: an evidence-based user's guide. Silver Spring, MD: US Food and Drug Administration, 2009.

[112] Minister of Health Canada. Strategic risk communications framework for Health Canada and the Public Health Agency of Canada. Ottawa: Minister of Health Canada, 2007. Accessible at: https://www.canada.ca/en/health-canada/corporate/about-health-canada/activities-responsibilities/risk-communications.html.

[113] Waisbord S, Larson H. Why Invest in communication for immunization: evidence and lessons learned. Baltimore, New York: Health Communication Partnership based at Johns Hopkins Bloomberg School of Public Health/Center for Communication Programs and the United Nations Children's Fund (UNICEF), 2005. Accessible at: http://www.who.int/immunization/hpv/communicate/why_invest_in_communication_for_immunization_unicef_healthcommunicationspartnership_path_usaid.pdf.

[114] Waisbord S, Larson H. Why invest in communication for immunization: evidence and lessons learned. Baltimore, New York: Health Communication Partnership based at Johns Hopkins Bloomberg School of Public Health, Center for Communication Programs and the United Nations Children's Fund (UNICEF), 2005. Accessible at: http://www.who.int/immunization/hpv/communicate/why_invest_in_communication_for_immunization_unicef_healthcommunicationspartnership_path_usaid.pdf.

[115] Karafillakis E, Larson H, on behalf of the ADVANCE consortium. A systematic literature review of perceived risks of vaccines in European populations. Vaccine. 2017; 35: 4840-4850..

[116] Waisbord S, Larson H., 2005.

[117] Based on: O'Sullivan GA, Yonkler JA, Morgan W, Merritt AP. A field guide to designing a health communication strategy. Baltimore, MD: Johns Hopkins Bloomberg School of Public Health, Center for Communication Programs: March 2003. Accessible at: http://ccp.jhu.edu/documents/A%20Field%20Guide%20to%20Designing%20Health%20Comm%20Strategy.pdf.

At the core of each VacSCP are its specific objectives in line with the overall aims of vaccine safety communication (see §2.2). According to the theory of the strategic approach to health communication, all concerned stakeholders should ideally work together and agree on the communication objectives, plan and materials. However, for a regulatory authority there is often little time to publish new data and the news cannot be shared preferentially with some groups prior to the general public. Yet to some extent multistakeholder collaboration is practiced; for a number of years in some jurisdictions regulatory authorities and the manufacturer have been agreeing on communication plans for interventions like direct healthcare professional communications (DHPCs) which have facilitated clarity and planning.[118, 119] There should also be agreement between regulatory authorities and the national immunization programmes, but it has to be understood that while the communication messages about the benefit-risk profile and safety of a vaccine should indeed be consistent, the communication plans will differ between these organizations, in order to align their objectives with the distinct mandates of each organization (i.e. marketing authorization of vaccine products and information about the benefit-risk balance versus issuance of vaccination schedules and promotion of vaccination for public health protection).

4.2. Developing VacSCPs on the basis of a model template

VacSCPs may be developed by the professionals of the vaccine safety communication system of the regulatory body (see §5.1) through a multistakeholder interaction (see §4.1 and §5.2), using the model template provided in Template 4.2.[120] This VacSCP model template is based on the communication plan template for vaccine safety events issued by WHO[121] and has been enhanced in line with the P-Process (see §4.1) and its application to pharmacovigilance.[122]

The effectiveness of a VacSCP will very much depend on the depth and width of the initial understanding of the situation and the audiences (see §2.1), and on the cooperation with stakeholders from the VacSCP development phase and the whole communication cycle (see §4.1). Guidance for understanding and monitoring the situation (which both use the same methods) is provided in §4.3.

---

[118] Following informal use for a number of years, the following template has been published as part of EU-GVP: European Medicines Agency (EMA) and Heads of Medicines Agencies. Guideline on good pharmacovigilance practices (GVP) – Annex II – Templates: Communication Plan for Direct Healthcare Professional Communication (CP DHPC). London: EMA, 8 December 2015, Rev 1 12 October 2017. Accessible at: http://www.ema.europa.eu/ema/index.jsp?curl=pages/regulation/document_listing/document_listing_000345.jsp&mid=WC0b01ac058058f32c.

[119] Health Canada. Issued Health Professional Communication - Dear Health Care Professional Letter document 3, 2008. http://www.hc-sc.gc.ca/dhp-mps/pubs/medeff/_guide/2008-risk-risques_comm_guid-dir/index-eng.php#Document3.

[120] The CIOMS VacSCP template is available in a downloadable form on the CIOMS website: www.cioms.ch.

[121] World Health Organization Regional Office for Europe. Vaccine safety events: managing the communications response. Copenhagen: WHO, 2013.

[122] Bahri P. Public pharmacovigilance communication: a process calling for evidence-based, objective-driven strategies. Drug Saf. 2010, 33: 1065-1079.

Template 4.2: Template for strategic vaccine type- and situation-specific vaccine safety communication plans (VacSCPs)

CIOMS Vaccine Safety Communication Plan (VacSCP)
Vaccine product(s): <insert names of concerned product(s)>

I. Situation and monitoring

Vaccine safety: <Describe briefly the benefit-risk profile of the vaccine(s), the use of the vaccine and its impact, and any safety concerns under surveillance, public debate or emerging.>

Epidemiology: <Describe key aspects and trends of disease epidemiology.>

Public: <Describe briefly the applicable considerations (see Chapter 2 of Guide) as well as other social and political considerations. Describe audiences and sub-audiences, their knowledge, attitudes and practices (KAP) and related concerns and information needs as well as media preferences. Describe stakeholders, including community/opinion leaders and cooperations. Describe the challenges and opportunities of communication in the given situation.>

Monitoring of public KAP, concerns, rumours and information needs: <Describe briefly monitoring activities to inform the VacSCP and keep it up-to-date during its development such as monitoring of the public debates in the media (using a defined list of media outlets to check daily, or using a media intelligence service or academic research departments), monitoring media queries and questions from the public to the organization, regular exchange with community/opinion leaders.>

II. Communication objectives

<Describe briefly which KAPs in the audiences (e.g. vaccination target population, their carers, healthcare professionals, policy makers, information multipliers) and health outcomes are intended to be achieved through communication, including through addressing public concerns and information needs. The objectives should be specific and measurable.>

III. Strategic design of the communication intervention

Target audiences: <Define and prioritize target audiences (e.g. the vaccination target population, their carers, healthcare professionals, policy makers, information multipliers (such as learned societies) and others) with specifying their sub-segments (e.g. by community, healthcare setting), including the audiences' barriers and facilitators for achieving the communication objectives. Describe how audiences can make their concerns made known to the organization and participate in the communication design process.>

Change model: <Define the motivating factors that are to be strengthened and mechanisms that may be applied to overcome barriers, both for achieving the communication objectives.>

Key messages: <Formulate short and understandable key messages on vaccine risks, safety and safe use behaviours with supporting facts tailored for each target (sub-) audience and define a mechanism for user-testing. Contextualise the safety concern with exposure data/ vaccination rates and the evidence on the benefit of the vaccine. Acknowledge public debate and concerns with respect and empathy.>

Communication tools and dissemination mechanisms in a mixed media approach: <Define the tools (e.g. written, visual or audio materials) to be used to carry the communication content and mechanisms to disseminate the content appropriate tailored to the target (sub-) audiences (e.g. printed materials to be handed out by healthcare provider, newsletter circulated by email or mobile to subscribers, article in a scientific journal or newspaper, community events, radio, television, website, social media platform).>

Interactions with journalists and community advocates/activists: <Establish information telephone lines or online tools for questions by the public and, if necessary, schedule press conferences. Prepare and annex to the VacSCP talking points for responding to queries from the media and others promptly.>

Timetable: <Schedule drafting, stakeholder consultation, user testing, finalization, (repeated) dissemination and evaluation of the communication interventions, and define who is responsible for which task by which date.>

Transparency provisions: <Note which background information will be published or made available to members of the public upon request and have them available (e.g. assessment reports).>

IV. Monitoring and evaluation

<Describe activities to monitor the dissemination and the intended and unintended impact of communication interventions, in particular the effectiveness in relation to the communication objectives, as well as any changes to the situation (e.g. the epidemiology of the disease to vaccinate against, public debate). Describe how the need, if identified by means of monitoring and evaluation, for improving communication and updating the VacSCP will be taken forward.>

A step-by-step guide to developing communication strategies for vaccine benefit-risk communication with practical examples has recently been developed in Europe and can also be helpful to follow when developing VacSCPs (see Guidance Summary 4.2).[123]

Guidance Summary 4.2: Developing communication strategies on vaccine benefits and risks

Communication strategies for vaccine benefit-risk information aims at maintaining and improve public confidence in vaccination by demonstrating that decisions about vaccination are based on robust data and integrity. It is therefore important to communicate about the partners generating and using data and their framework of collaboration, including their code of conduct and quality management processes.[124]

The development of such communication strategies should follow a practical stepwise approach:

- ▶ Step 1: define goals and objectives of the communication strategy;
- ▶ Step 2: map and engage with the various stakeholders;

---

[123] Accelerated Development of Vaccine beNefit-risk Collaboration in Europe (ADVANCE). Developing Communication Strategies on Vaccine Benefits and Risks. ADVANCE, 2017. Available at: http://www.advance-vaccines.eu/?page=publications&id=DELIVERABLES.

[124] Accelerated Development of Vaccine beNefit-risk Collaboration in Europe (ADVANCE). Developing Communication Strategies on Vaccine Benefits and Risks. ADVANCE, 2017. Available at: http://www.advance-vaccines.eu/?page=publications&id=DELIVERABLES.

> ▶ Step 3: develop the communication content and core components of the strategy (e.g. selected audiences, preferred channels) (step 3);
>
> ▶ Step 4: plan implementation and monitoring. (step 4).

4.3. Monitoring, evaluating and maintaining VacSCPs

The VacSCP is a 'living document' to be updated to meet changing situations: New risks or safety information may emerge at any time during the life-cycle of a vaccine (see Chapter 3), the epidemiology of the disease to vaccinate against may change over time as well as the public KAP, concerns and information needs. Among other things, the public debate overall may increase, decrease or change in focus or stakeholders involved.

Therefore regular monitoring and evaluation activities are necessary to maintain the VacSCP and adapt it at any time before, during and after a communication intervention. When deciding on revising or designing future communication interventions and their timings, stakeholders need to take into account the risk of either over-communication and related the amplification of risk perception (see §2.2) or alert fatigue and associated decrease in risk perception and adherence to safe use advice.[125] Real-time monitoring and regular evaluation, and subsequent adjustments are also essential for preventing and managing crisis situations.

In addition VacSCPs need to be updated with the learnings from the evaluation of the communication intervention as part of the cyclic communication process (see §4.1). The evaluation is a 'lessons learnt' exercise, describing the effectiveness of the communication intervention in relation to the set objectives, or unintended effects, whether positive or negative. More specifically, the purpose of evaluation is to identify further communication needs for maintaining or improving success, and to adjust the VacSCP and communication interventions, building on the experience and evidence generated by the evaluation.

Evaluating communication interventions and thereby the vaccine communication system (see Chapter 5) forms part of quality management of the system and is necessary for fulfilling accountability through evidence. This should contribute to justifying resources for vaccine safety communication systems. Evaluating is not an easy task, but it is essential for the sustainability of the systems and their outcomes. However, rather than looking at evaluation from a sequential process perspective only, a broader view incorporates a continuous real-time monitoring of the implementation and impact of communication interventions in addition to evaluations after an intervention.

The methods and results of monitoring and evaluating of implementation, its effectiveness and other impact should be transparent and explained in their meaning and limitations. The main challenge lies in finding methods and meaningful indicators, which ideally can, beyond describing change, also study causal relationships with the communication interventions and the factors which may influence impact. For this, data pre- and post-intervention as well as on influences other than the intervention should be collected. In any case one should ensure that mechanisms are in place for simple monitoring and feedback from all audiences. These may include measuring the dissemination of messages through various media, KAP surveys, media monitoring and calculating vaccination rates. The acronym KAP provides a reminder to conduct surveys comprehensively, to capture knowledge, attitude and practice.[126]

---

[125] Agency for Healthcare Quality and Research (AHQR), U.S. Department of Health and Human Services. Patient safety primer: alert fatigue. Rockville, MD: AHQR, June 2017. Accessible at: https://psnet.ahrq.gov/primers/primer/28/alert-fatigue.

[126] United Nations Children's Fund Regional Office for South Asia (UNICEF-ROSA). Building trust and responding to adverse events following immunisation in South Asia: using strategic communication. Kathmandu: UNICEF-ROSA, 2005.

In relation to knowledge, it should be measured how far an audience's awareness and understanding of factual information has changed. Through attitude surveys, one can study the sentiments people have formed about something or somebody, and how these change over time (e.g. from hostile to neutral or accepting of a proposal like vaccination or safe use advice, or to becoming increasingly adverse and non-trusting). Practice relates to the behaviour, such as actual vaccination.

4.3.1 Monitoring of debates and sentiments in communities and the public

Monitoring of the public debates in the news and/or social media can happen daily using a defined list of newspapers in paper or online news media outlets, social media search tools, or through making use of a media intelligence service[127] or academic research departments. The feasibility and usefulness of media monitoring is illustrated with examples from the polio immunization program in Israel (see Example 4.3.1) and from the European Medicines Agency (EMA) for a safety assessment on HPV vaccines (see Example 4.3.2). A good example for monitoring Twitter for vaccine debates in multiple languages can be found in the literature.[128] One can also monitor media queries and questions from the public to the organization. Regular exchange with community and opinion leaders can also provide important insights, and supplement quantitative data (i.e. obtained through measurement) with regard to possible causal relationships and factors influencing communication effectiveness. Where measurements are difficult, the observations from community and opinion leaders able to provide feedback in comprehensive, unbiased manner are even more valuable.

---

[127] This may be a commercial service, but non-commercial tools are also available for own use, such as MEDISYS, provided by the European Commission under: https://ec.europa.eu/jrc/en/scientific-tool/medical-information-system.

[128] Becker BF, Larson HJ, Bonhoeffer J, van Mulligen EM, Sturkenboom MC. Evaluation of a multinational, multilingual vaccine debate on Twitter. Vaccine. 2016; 34: 6166-6171.

Example 4.3.1: Social media monitoring during polio supplementary immunization activities (SIA) in Israel

In response to the reintroduction of wild poliovirus, the Israeli Ministry of Health, in 2013, conducted a large-scale media campaign with successful media monitoring. In that year, a wild poliovirus was detected in routine environmental surveillance in a sewage system in the Southern part of Israel. The population immunity was high, with vaccination coverage with inactivated polio vaccine (IPV) above 95% and without detection of actual polio-cases. Still, it was decided to implement supplementary immunization activities (SIA) with oral and injected polio vaccines.

Initially, this decision caused resistance in some groups. However, through concerted effort and a comprehensive communication strategy the campaign became a success. A key element contributing to this success was a sophisticated system of media monitoring to understand public opinion and respond to concerns. As part of this effort, health authorities via social media became aware of a planned anti-vaccination protest demonstration and were able to mobilize polio victims to address the public at this demonstration. An indication of the success of the campaign is that at the beginning only 55% of parents said they would bring their children for supplementary immunization, but a few months later, after the communication interventions, 75% of the targeted children had been vaccinated, i.e. more than 900,000 out of 1.2 million.[129]

Example 4.3.2: Utility of online news media monitoring for prepared communicating of the outcome of a safety assessment for HPV vaccines at the European Medicines Agency (EMA)

Public debate regularly centers around the benefit-risk of vaccines often taking place in traditional and social media. To address this trend, the European Medicines Agency (EMA) wanted to examine the utility of media monitoring and how it could be useful for regulatory bodies. In 2015 EMA conducted a media monitoring study concerning human papillomavirus (HPV) vaccines over the period of time during which a procedure was instigated to investigate the potential causality of two suspected adverse reactions reported to the authorities: complex regional pain syndrome (CRPS) and postural orthostatic tachycardia syndrome (POTS).

Prospective real-time monitoring of worldwide online news was undertaken from September to December 2015 with inductive content analysis. More than 4000 news items - originals and re-posted ones - were collected, containing personal stories, scientific and policy/process-related topics. Explicit and implicit concerns voiced in the news media and some linked blogs were identified, including those raised due to lack of knowledge or anticipated once more information would be published, generating 'derived questions'.

Rather than describing these concerns and information needs in factual style, those collected until 24 October were 'translated' into scientific or regulatory language and formulated as 50 questions (which could be categorized into 12 themes). The questions related to a wide range of topics, such as CRPS and POTS case definitions, underreporting of suspected adverse reactions, trustworthiness of data as well as the standards and code of conducts of regulatory bodies.

---

[129] Kaliner E, Moran-Gilad J, Grotto I, et al. Silent reintroduction of wild-type poliovirus to Israel, 2013: risk communication challenges in an argumentative atmosphere. Euro Surveill. 2014, 19: 20703.

The 'derived questions' were provided to assessors and medical writers/media officers at the EMA and the EU member states for use in real life and preparing the communication of the outcome of the assessment on 5 November. It was demonstrated that providing media monitoring findings to assessors and medical writers/media officers resulted in: (1) confirming that public concerns regarding CRPS and POTS would be covered by the assessment; (2) meeting specific information needs proactively in the public statement; (3) predicting all queries from journalists received at the press conference on 5 November and in writing thereafter; and (4) altering the tone of the public statement with respectful acknowledgement of the health status of CRSP and POTS patients.

The study demonstrated the utility of media monitoring for regulatory bodies to support communication proactivity and preparedness. Derived questions seem to be a suitable method since regulators normally formulate situations as research questions. Presenting media monitoring results in the scientific-regulatory environment and formulating the media content as questions were both novel approaches that yielded useful information. The study suggests that media monitoring could form part of regular surveillance for medicines of high public interest.[130]

---

[130] Bahri P, Fogd J, Morales D, Kurz X, ADVANCE consortium. Application of real-time global media monitoring and 'derived questions' for enhancing communication by regulatory bodies: the case of human papillomavirus vaccines. BMC Medicine. 2017 May 2, 15:91.

CHAPTER 5.
VACCINE SAFETY COMMUNICATION SYSTEMS

5.1. Functions of vaccine safety communication systems

Generally, systems are understood as consisting of structures and processes to fulfil certain objectives; and in order to enable preparing and implementing planned communication, a vaccine safety communication system consists of certain key functions (see Checklist 5.1). Depending on the structure of the regulatory authority, all functions might form one dedicated department or there might be a split between planning, implementing and evaluating communication interventions. Taking into account local resources, opportunities and priorities, an organization may choose which functions to build up first and to which extent, so that a tailored system can be built up over time.

Checklist 5.1: Key functions of vaccine safety communication systems

- ☑ Development of strategic vaccine-type and situation-specific vaccine safety communication plans (VacSCPs)
- ☑ Establishment and maintenance of multistakeholder networks
- ☑ Collaboration at local, country, regional and international level
- ☑ Monitoring of vaccine knowledge, attitudes, practices (KAP) and related concerns, rumours and information needs
- ☑ Interaction with the media through a dedicated spokesperson
- ☑ Development of communication messages and materials
- ☑ Implementation of communication interventions
- ☑ Evaluation of communication interventions
- ☑ Management of vaccine safety crisis

5.2. Multistakeholder network

Vaccine safety communication consists of complex processes of listening and messaging between those with responsibilities for vaccine safety as well as institutional and public stakeholders at local, country, regional and international level (see Table 5.2.1).

Table 5.2.1: Main stakeholders involved in the vaccine safety communication process

- Regulatory authorities
- Public health authorities
- National immunization committees
- National advisory committees on adverse events following immunization
- Health technology assessment bodies
- Ministries of health
- Local and national politicians
- Vaccine manufacturers
- Representatives of vaccine target populations, vaccinees, parents, carers and the community (villages, civil society), including e.g. women's groups, anti-vaccine groups, citizen watchdogs
- Religious and community/public opinion leaders, including e.g. teachers
- Representatives from healthcare professionals in public and private healthcare, traditional and alternative healer communities, healthcare professional associations, learned societies
- Media representatives and journalists
- Non-governmental organizations
- Donors and procurement agencies
- Technical development agencies
- Multilateral agencies, e.g. World Health Organization (WHO) and its Global Advisory Committee on Vaccine Safety (GACVS), UNICEF

Any stakeholder group or individual may take particular roles in shaping public and personal sentiments and impact on knowledge, attitude and behaviour of individuals. Opinion leaders may be healthcare, community and religious leaders, teachers, journalists, or come from a trusted governmental or non-governmental organization or interest groups like anti-vaccine groups, women's groups or citizen watchdog groups. An opinion leader can come from inside or outside a concerned community or country. Opinion leaders may specifically act as intermediaries between the authorities and the public. Communication in the public domain impacts on interpersonal communication between individuals in healthcare settings as it occurs (e.g. when discussing informed consent, proposed vaccination of children or suspected harm due to a vaccine). Individuals often trust their physician, nurse, midwife, pharmacist and/or other traditional/alternative healthcare professionals or sources.

An essential function of a vaccine safety communication system therefore is the stakeholder and community network, which needs to be established over time and be carefully maintained (see Checklist 5.2) for a number of important objectives (see Table 5.2.2). Overall, collaboration with the network should allow for multiple perspectives on vaccines and approaches to solve issues, making use of communication for increasing common understanding, disseminating the evidence base and achieving agreements. Understanding of the complexity of the network may be facilitated by thinking about and mapping interactions according the social ecological model (SEM)(see §2.1).

Checklist 5.2: Establishing and maintaining national stakeholder networks

- ☑ Set objectives of interactions
- ☑ Build capacity and infrastructure for public dialogue and deliberation
- ☑ Map majority and minority stakeholders, their roles and how to approach them, including in case of vaccine or communication crisis

- ☑ Create a national media map
- ☑ Define mechanisms and policies for interactions
- ☑ Establish a code of conduct for governmental organizations and other policies to avoid lobbying, conflict of interests and bias and keep transparency
- ☑ Demand, as a governmental organization, transparency from all stakeholders of information sources, finances and interests
- ☑ Define a policy for what are appropriate collaborations from vaccine manufacturers
- ☑ Create a public calendar of interactions, e.g. newsletters and events
- ☑ Publish outcomes of interactions and express thanks for the contributions
- ☑ Offer subscriptions and services to ask questions and provide feedback

Table 5.2.2: Purposes of multistakeholder interactions

- ▸ Listening to current understanding, concerns and information needs of the public regarding vaccines in general and in relation to specific issues;
- ▸ Involvement of audiences in the development of VacSCPs and communication interventions, including usability testing;
- ▸ Provision of collaboration, e.g. for defining and agreeing messages about vaccine risks/safety, participation of community(ies) in consultations undertaken by regulatory authorities and deliberation processes;
- ▸ Interactions with the media; and
- ▸ Demonstrating trustworthiness and trust-building.

The institutional stakeholders at local and country level include those in charge of vaccine licensure, healthcare payments and reimbursement, procurement, supply management, immunization policy-making and immunization program management. Also, stakeholders along the vaccine supply chains may need to communicate at population level, as they have the responsibility for selecting high quality safe vaccines and distributing them safely. Vaccine manufacturers are an institutional stakeholder too, and may be from inside or outside the country. Each of the institutions will have their assigned responsibility in the overall vaccine safety process within the country and consequently have a need for their own vaccine safety communication systems. Communication between these institutional parties may or may not happen in the public domain.

Mechanisms need to be in place for cooperation between these organizations, so that communication messages about the safety of specific vaccines are consistent, despite that communication objectives will differ between organizations in accordance with their legal mandate. For example, public health agencies have to primarily communicate about the immunization programmes, while regulatory authorities communicate about the benefit-risk profiles of individual vaccine products. Despite close collaboration, regulatory authorities and other public bodies must keep their independence. Likewise the legal responsibilities of all parties in vaccine safety have to be respected as well as the independence of the media.

Public stakeholders include the vaccine target populations, their families, healthcare professionals, the communities, interest groups and the media. The media are comprised of both traditional and evolving print, paper, mail, poster, television, radio, electronic and web-based news and social media, such as Facebook and Twitter. Interactions with the media should provide journalists, proactively and in responsively, with accurate information about the safety profile and safe use of vaccines, without trying to influence them in a way that would, truly or be perceived as, trying to jeopardize the independence and freedom of the media.

Good interaction with stakeholders can prevent a crisis situation, as shown in the following Example 5.2.

Example 5.2: Managing an adverse event following immunization with HPV vaccine in the United Kingdom

In September 2008, the Department of Health (DH) of the United Kingdom (UK) launched their national programme to vaccinate girls aged 12-13 against human papillomavirus (HPV). At the same time, a two-year catch-up campaign began to vaccinate older girls under the age of 18 years. The programme has largely been delivered through secondary schools. Three doses of HPV vaccine are given over a six-month period. The first year of the programme achieved high vaccination coverage with all three doses (81% of the girls aged 12-13 years).[131] More than 1.4 million doses had been given since the vaccination programme started.

On 28 September 2009, a 14-year old girl died shortly after receiving an HPV vaccination at her school in Coventry, UK. When a serious adverse event following immunization (AEFI) occurs, it is important that accurate information is communicated in the media and that the facts of the event do not become distorted. Through proper handling of the media response to AEFIs, health officials can avoid loss of public confidence in vaccination. The following table summarizes the events of 2008 and how the respective authorities responded as the events unfolded:

Day 1 - September 28, 2009	
Student dies 75 minutes after HPV vaccination.	Known medical facts: • 10:45 a 14-year old girl receives an HPV vaccination along with other girls in her school. • At about 11:30 she collapses at school. • By noon she has died at the hospital. • There was no evidence of an acute allergic reaction.
Responses	
Local health department (NHS Coventry)	1. Informed the UK DH immunization director. 2. Informed the national drug regulator (MHRA) of an adverse event through the yellow card system. 3. Issued a brief press statement including facts of death, sympathies to family and friends, and announcing that an urgent and full investigation was being conducted. Statement also warned that: "No link can be made between the death and the vaccine until all the facts are known and a post mortem takes place."

---

[131] United Kingdom Department of Health and Health Protection Agency. Annual HPV vaccine uptake in England 2008/09.

National health department (UK DH)	1. Quarantined vaccine batch as a precautionary measure and alerted local Directors of Public Health, Immunisation Coordinators and General Practitioners. 2. Confirmed that MHRA had received yellow card and began investigation. 3. Issued press statement with facts of death and information on the vaccination programme. 4. Decided not to suspend vaccination programme during the investigation. 5. Decided not to assign a government spokesperson for interview requests. 6. Decided not to make any further statements until new information was available.
School misinforms parents	Sent a letter to parents that said: "An unfortunate incident occurred and one of the girls suffered a rare, but extreme reaction to the vaccine." However, at this point the cause of death was unknown and it was impossible to say whether this tragedy was caused by a reaction to the vaccine. Even though the school corrected this information on their website later that evening, it caused confusion and concern among the parents and media.
High media interest	Local and international evening broadcast news reports girl's death shortly after receiving HPV vaccination. High interest from media in the story.

Day 2 - September 29	
Responses	
Political opposition criticizes government	An opposition politician noted that the government had chosen the vaccine product used and suggested that the competitor's vaccine could have been a safer option. He called for safety data to be published.
Manufacturer recalls vaccine batch	Manufacturer voluntarily recalled vaccine batch.
National (UK DH) waits for new information	Decided not to respond to political opposition claims and followed their policy against making additional statements until new information was available. There was concern it could be days before the autopsy results were known. Internal intelligence allowed communications offers to brief journalists with whom they had a relationship to be cautious about any speculation that the vaccine caused the death until more information was known.
Preliminary post-mortem results	In the evening, preliminary autopsy results found that the girl's death was due to a rare serious underlying medical condition and that the vaccination did not play a role in her death.

UK DH contacts media	At about 9:30 PM UK DH communication officers urgently began contacting TV news teams, followed by the Press Association, and newspapers in time for the 10 PM UK television news programmes, and to reverse any negative headlines in the next day's papers.
High media interest	Interest in story remains high. Evening broadcast news (10 PM) reported preliminary post-mortem results.

Day 3 - September 30
Responses

UK National Institute for Biological Standards and Control	Preliminary testing of vaccine batch found it to fully conform to all safety standards.
National (UK DH)	Informed school services to continue immunizing with HPV vaccine. Offered government spokespeople for interviews with the media, but media was no longer interested.
Secondary story emerges....	Legal firm alerted the press that it was representing the families of 10 English girls who, they claim, had been adversely affected by HPV vaccination. It is the basis for two features, one in the Daily Mail, the other in Sunday Times.
Media	Most morning newspapers did not reflect preliminary post-mortem results. Preliminary post-mortem results announced during the day. Story begins to die out in the mainstream press.

Day 4 - October 1
Responses

Post-mortem results published	Preliminary post-mortem results are published.
National (UK DH) reaches out to media	Offered government spokespeople for interviews with the media, but there is little interest from the media.
Media coverage drops	Reports on published post-mortem results. Story continues to die out in the mainstream press.

The death of the student shortly following HPV vaccination instigated widespread media attention, sometimes with erroneous, misleading, confusing headlines, and provoked public concern about the vaccine. Some media stories created a false assumption that there was a true risk with the vaccine. Some stories created the impression that the vaccination programme was in chaos, and by implication that the government had lost control of the situation.

The most vivid example of inaccurate reporting was published in the weekly Sunday Express on 4 October ("Jab as deadly as the cancer"), eight days after the student's death and long after the vaccine was cleared from playing a role in the death. Independent news media plays a pivotal role shaping public perception of vaccination programmes. In this case, the media was most interested in the story when there were unanswered questions about the safety of the vaccine. These kinds of questions can give rise to rumours and false information. It is therefore important for vaccine safety communicators to get in front of the story to frame the questions in the media and provide accurate answers rather than be reactive because chasing and countering rumours and misinformation is difficult and often not entirely successful.

The HPV vaccination programme in the UK was not at any point in time in jeopardy. In Coventry, the local National Health Service (NHS) did not suspend its vaccination programme, but rescheduled clinics for Tuesday and Wednesday to give staff the chance to be fully briefed to answer public enquiries. In some areas vaccination sessions were temporarily halted because their vaccine supply was from the batch that was quarantined.

This case never reached crisis level due to the immediate and appropriate management of the situation by the UK DH.

The following contributed in particular to this effective management:

- Immediate coordination of communications with school officials;
- Issuing of a preliminary statement within a few hours;
- Close collaboration between government communication and immunization departments;
- Being careful about making public comments when not yet fully informed and confirming available facts before making any public statements;
- Communication with receptive journalists with whom a relationship already exists;
- Keeping politics out of the story;
- Being sensitive (while the administration of a vaccine shortly before this girl died was a coincidence, all correspondence needed to be sensitive to the fact that this was a local tragedy).

Immediate management requires being prepared, especially regarding the following:

- Knowing the baseline incidence of possible serious adverse events;
- Training vaccination personnel at all levels to respond adequately;
- Prepare a plan to react to a crisis when it occurs, including immediate reporting of AEFIs to the national agency responsible for pharmacovigilance.

With a view to understand the impact of the student's death on the public perception of HPV vaccines and thereby also evaluate the impact of the communication during the investigations, the UK DH designed a survey that would allow them to compare current public perceptions with those existing before the programme began. They could do so because the UK DH had conducted surveys, beginning three years before the introduction of HPV vaccination, as follows:

- 2005. Initial qualitative research conducted among parents about their attitudes and awareness of HPV and HPV vaccine.
- 2007. Just over a year before the launch of the programme, surveys were carried out among students, parents and health professionals:

- one survey measured the opinions of HPV vaccination among parents of 8- 9 years-old girls;
  - this survey was repeated among 12-years-old girls and their parents;
  - this information was intended to determine the most acceptable age to target vaccination, as it was important programmatically because it shifted the implementation from primary to secondary school environments;
  - Some of these surveys provided "pre-campaign" or "baseline" data to be used to monitor changes in attitudes and awareness of HPV vaccine.
- 2008. Once the vaccination programme was underway – the routine programme began as well as the catch-up campaign – surveys were regularly carried out to track progress and detect changes in the programme.
- 2009-10. Surveys were regularly carried out to track progress and detect changes in the programme, while the routine programme continued and the catch-up campaign was concluded.

Further in 2007 a survey measured public perception of the vaccine by asking mothers and daughters to read an information card on HPV and the vaccination programme. They were then asked how favourable they felt towards the vaccination. In that survey at least four out of five respondents (80%) in each group said they were "very" or "fairly" favourable of the HPV vaccine. After the death of the student, the UK HD conducted a new survey, again asking mothers and daughters to read an information card on HPV and the vaccination programme and how favourable they felt towards the vaccine. There were no significant changes in the high levels of favourability toward the HPV vaccine after the student's death. At least four out of five respondents (80%) in each group said they were "very" or "fairly" favourable of the HPV vaccine.

The awareness that a student had died shortly after receiving HPV vaccination was assessed by an additional survey. Mothers and daughters were asked what they had recently seen or heard in the media about HPV. Between two and three in ten mentioned the event in their responses (i.e. they demonstrated spontaneous awareness). If the student death was not mentioned at this stage, respondents were asked directly if they were aware of the incident – this question measured prompted awareness. Including prompted responses, over 80% of mothers and 70% of daughters were aware of the case. The remaining mothers and daughters were "not aware" of the incident.

Those who had reported being aware of the death of the student were asked to describe how concerned they had initially felt at the time the event occurred. At least seven in ten of respondents were initially concerned about the vaccine. When mothers and daughters were asked how concerned they currently felt, now that it was clear that the girl's death was not linked to the HPV vaccination, most mothers and daughters were no longer concerned about the HPV vaccine.

Today, the UK regularly monitors public opinion on vaccination and trust in health authorities through both quantitative and qualitative research. This means that they are able to detect changes in public trust or opinions on vaccination and respond to them, long before they could develop into a crisis. [132]

---

[132] World Health Organization (WHO). Managing an adverse event following immunization: an interactive case study. Geneva: WHO, 2011. Accessible at: http://vaccine-safety-training.org/c-resources.html.

5.3. Regional and international awareness and collaboration

Immunization is a matter of global public health and news and rumours may travel quickly. For these reasons, a vaccine safety communication system needs to maintain awareness of the vaccine safety-related discussions around the globe that may have an impact in one's own country. On particular issues, an adverse event reported in one country may have implications for other places using the same product or batch of a particular vaccine. Optimal international communication on vaccine safety issues can be enhanced when those national authorities in charge of the national immunization program or assessment and licensure of vaccines, that are the main government entities responsible for vaccine safety, are familiar with international parties and experts who can provide them with information, independent advice or information to rely upon for key messages. In Figure 5.3 the relationships between the main parties for global collaboration are presented. This schematic highlights the need for the stakeholder network (see §5.2.) not only to cover the local or country level, but also to enable regional and international collaboration.

Figure 5.3: Relationships of parties in global vaccine safety

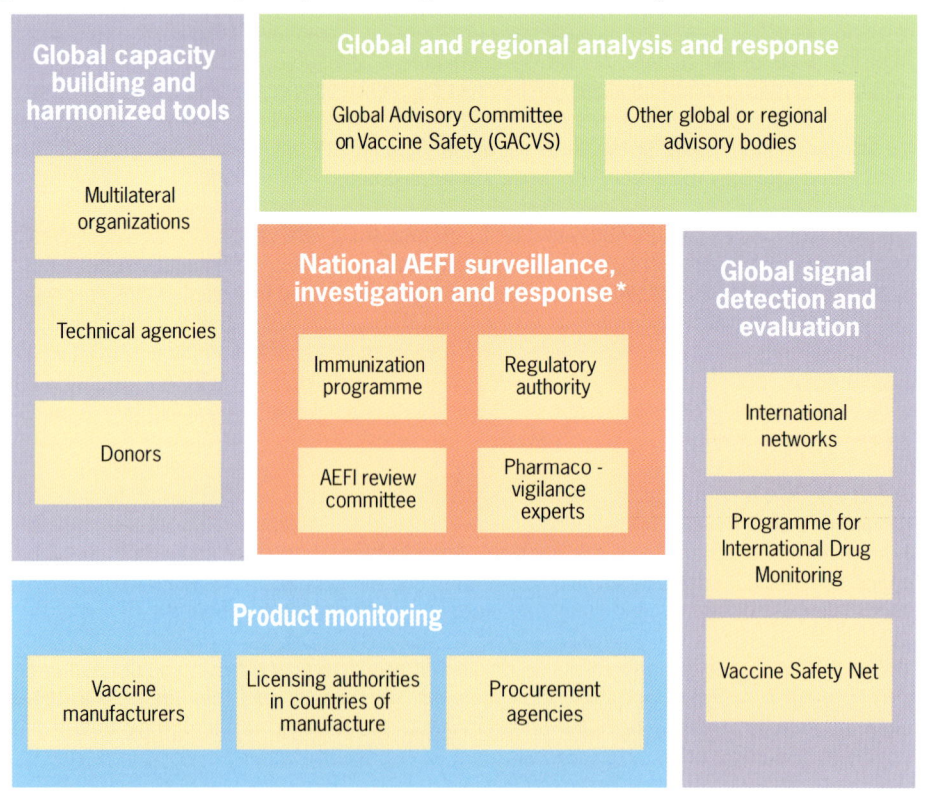

Global capacity building and harmonized tools
- Multilateral organizations
- Technical agencies
- Donors

Global and regional analysis and response
- Global Advisory Committee on Vaccine Safety (GACVS)
- Other global or regional advisory bodies

National AEFI surveillance, investigation and response*
- Immunization programme
- Regulatory authority
- AEFI review committee
- Pharmaco-vigilance experts

Global signal detection and evaluation
- International networks
- Programme for International Drug Monitoring
- Vaccine Safety Net

Product monitoring
- Vaccine manufacturers
- Licensing authorities in countries of manufacture
- Procurement agencies

* Several entities that participate in the national primary health care system usually contribute to vaccine pharmacovigilance.

Source: World Health Organization. Adapted for CIOMS Guide to Active Vaccine Safety Surveillance, 2017.[133]

---

[133] World Health Organization. Adapted for CIOMS Guide to Active Vaccine Safety Surveillance (2017) from graphic WHO entitled, "Components of a 21st Century global vaccine safety monitoring, investigation, and response system." Module 5: Vaccine safety institutions and mechanisms Vaccine safety basics learning manual, www.vaccine-safety-training.org.

At international level, a number of stakeholders are specifically important for LMICs: The Global Advisory Committee on Vaccine Safety (GACVS) provides independent, authoritative, scientific advice to WHO on vaccine safety issues of global or regional concerns with the potential to affect in the short or long term national immunization programmes. Its assessments of vaccine safety issues are publicly available and statements are occasionally produced when urgent concerns are identified.[134] WHO Strategic Advisory Group of Experts (SAGE) develops recommendations for vaccine utilization based on a risk-benefit analysis informed by GACVS assessments. WHO, UNICEF and their country offices and other partner technical agencies and donors are engaged in the Global Vaccine Safety Initiative (GVSI). Donors are important parties as they interact with immunization policy decision-makers, can prioritize resources, and provide access to non-state and private sector parties.

Particularly for supporting communication a country level, WHO has created the Vaccine Safety Net (VSN) [135] as a network of more than forty reputable governmental, professional associations and academic websites (with a combined reach estimated at millions of visits each year) that provide vaccine safety information in various languages. Each website has been evaluated by WHO and after having met criteria for good information practices was added to the VSN list of reliable websites. The VSN aims to address the variable reliability of information available from the worldwide web. This is particularly relevant in the area of vaccine safety, where a high number of websites provide incomplete or misleading information, including unfounded rumours or fraudulent research. This can lead to undue fears und uncertainties among the general public and undermine immunization programmes.

The Uppsala Monitoring Centre[136] maintains for the WHO Programme for International Drug Monitoring, a global data base of individual case safety reports, called VigiBase, which can be accessed by member countries of the programme in order to verify if similar issues have been identified elsewhere with a particular vaccine product.

---

[134] World Health Organization (WHO). Global Advisory Committee on Vaccine Safety (GACVS) [website]. Accessible at: http://www.who.int/vaccine_safety/initiative/communication/network/_gacvs/en/.

[135] World Health Organization (WHO). Vaccine safety net. Accessible at: http://www.who.int/vaccine_safety/initiative/communication/network/vaccine_safety_websites/en/.

[136] Uppsala Monitoring Centre https://www.who-umc.org/

CHAPTER 6.
CAPACITY BUILDING FOR VACCINE SAFETY COMMUNICATION SYSTEMS

6.1. Skills and capacity requirements

People working on vaccine safety communication require a set of critical skills and capacities (see Checklist 6.1). The communication system needs to support the application of these skills with appropriate structures and processes within the organization. More than one person may be required to cover all what is required, and a team will be needed in large organizations. In addition to technical communication skills, the overall mind set and empathy as well as emotional and relationship intelligence are specifically crucial for anybody working vaccine safety communication, requiring qualities of imagination, openness and appropriate behaviours. Empathy is the ability to understand and share the feelings of another;[137] this must be based on knowledge of what individuals or groups are thinking and feeling. No communication or information, however creative, colourful or modern, will reach and influence audiences unless this essential understanding and connection is made. The connection is supported through research, engagement and dialogue with the audiences.

Checklist 6.1: Skills and capacity requirements for vaccine safety communication

- ☑ Alert, listening, agile and responsive mind set
- ☑ Sensitive, contextualizing, far-seeing and proactive approach
- ☑ Understanding of the communication sciences and operations for an overall professional approach
- ☑ Ability to develop and apply quality management to communication processes
- ☑ Decision-making and implementation abilities
- ☑ Ability to establish and maintain strong, honest and trusted networks at community, expert and policy levels
- ☑ Knowledge and understanding of the medical and scientific issues as well as the social, political, economic, religious and cultural issues, and of how these issues affect risk perceptions and vaccination decisions in different groups
- ☑ Skills in reviewing and interpreting media debates
- ☑ Empathy and the ability to tailor messages meeting the audiences' differential needs in terms of information content, presentation and tone,
- ☑ Ability to act in ways that show the audiences that they are understood and taken seriously
- ☑ Ability to communicate in a clear, honest and transparent manner at eye level with the people and communities addressed

---

[137] Oxford Dictionary. Accessible at https://en.oxforddictionaries.com/definition/empathy, Accessed on 10 November 2016.

- ☑ Knowledge of information technology, keeping up with developments of new and social media and 'big data' in terms of technology and their use by the different audiences
- ☑ Ability to prevent and manage crisis situations
- ☑ Ability to evaluate and judge the effectiveness of communication interventions with a view to continuous improvement

Source: Bruce Hugman, Consultant, Uppsala Monitoring Centre.[138]

6.2. Contents and objectives of training

The structure of training events for vaccine safety communication systems can be based on the modular curriculum for teaching pharmacovigilance, issued jointly by WHO and the International Society of Pharmacovigilance (ISoP), which contains a module on communication. This module recommends teaching content in four areas that can be filled with vaccine-specific training content. (see Table 6.2).[139] Training courses should also be adapted to different and emerging vaccine safety situations, and be tailored to the needs of the participants and their different roles.

Table 6.2: Curriculum for vaccine safety communication

Area (WHO-ISOP)	Topics (adapted from WHO-ISOP)
1. Context and guidance	Public health goals, immunization policies, life-cycle safety management of vaccines, vaccine sentiments, cognitive concepts, guidance documents relevant to vaccine safety communication, vaccine safety communication systems, communication plans, crisis prevention and management, legal considerations, skills requirements
2. Communication with patients and healthcare professionals: tools, channels and processes	Individual and mass communication, participation of the public, tools and channels for listening/understanding audiences, messaging and obtaining feedback data for evaluation
3. Communication with patients and healthcare professionals: contents and presentation	Tailoring for target populations, including parents, selection and presentation of data, information elements and structure of the text, typical (tested) subject-matters and recommendations
4. Interaction among stakeholders including the media	Communication for involvement of the stakeholders in pharmacovigilance processes and communication planning, interaction with scientific and general media, press conferencing interactions between parties for evaluating communication

---

[138] Hugman B. Expecting the worst. Uppsala: Uppsala Monitoring Centre; 2010.

[139] Beckmann J, Hagemann U, Bahri P, Bate A, Boyd IW, Dal Pan GJ, Edwards BD, Edwards IR, Hartigan-Go K, Lindquist M, McEwen J, Moride Y, Olsson S, Pal SN, Soulaymani-Bencheikh R, Tuccori M, Vaca CP, Wong IC. Teaching pharmacovigilance: the WHO-ISoP core elements of a comprehensive modular curriculum. Drug Saf. 2014, 37:743–759.

Training should enable the participants to:

- understand the specificities of communicating on vaccine benefit-risk profiles, vaccine licensure and launch, routine immunization, mass immunization campaigns and public health emergencies;
- define communication objectives and desired outcomes;
- engage with and analyse audiences;
- develop strategic vaccine safety communication plans;
- interact efficiently with colleagues specialized in information technology;
- communicate in practice, including in crisis situations;
- confidently deal with the media.

Trainings should share knowledge and develop skills through plenary presentations, facilitated discussions, case-based group work, practical tasks and simulation exercises of real life situations. Innovative learning methods should be used, as they may be developed in the future. Accessing and using reliable vaccine safety information efficiently needs to be practiced too. The Vaccine Safety Net of WHO is one information major source for public health authorities, health professionals and the public.[140] Interpersonal communication skills need to be addressed as a key skill in all areas of vaccine safety communication. During training, national communication policies and processes may be tested and improved.

Example 6.2.1: Training programme on vaccine safety communication by the WHO Regional Office for Europe (WHO-EURO)

An exclusive vaccine safety communication course has been developed by the WHO Regional Office for Europe to improve the capacity, quality and effectiveness of communication responses to vaccine safety-related events with a focus on improving decision-making, response time and quality in responding to these events, including situations where real or perceived adverse events are affecting trust and confidence. The training programme draws on evidence from social psychology and communication science as well as case examples and lessons learned in countries.[141]

Example 6.2.2: Training resources of the Network for Education and Support in Immunisation (NESI)

The Network for Education and Support in Immunisation (NESI) was officially launched on 1 September 2002. NESI was built on the experience of the International Network for Eastern and Southern Africa on Hepatitis B Vaccination, which was established in 1999 and included five universities in Eastern and Southern Africa (Kenya, Tanzania, Zambia, Zimbabwe and South Africa), Ministries of Health in Africa and the University of Antwerp. The purpose of this network was to translate research on hepatitis B through capacity building and advocacy into universal access to hepatitis B vaccination in the partner countries.

---

[140] WHO Vaccine Safety Net. Accessible at: http://www.who.int/vaccine_safety/initiative/communication/network/vaccine_safety_websites/en/.

[141] The theoretical background and the stepwise guidance are available in the WHO-EURO 'vaccination and trust' online library: euro.who.int/vaccinetrust.

With the development of new vaccines and increased commitment by development partners and private sector initiatives to strengthen vaccine supply and immunization services, there are more opportunities to prevent additional diseases in larger numbers of infants, children, adolescents and adults. This led to the establishment of NESI, which is a collaborative network focusing on capacity building for the strengthening of existing immunization systems and introduction of new vaccines, with a broad technical scope and wide geographical focus.[142]

6.3. Comprehensive approach to capacity building

In general, capacity building has been defined as the creation of an enabling environment with appropriate policy and legal frameworks, institutional development, including community participation (of women in particular), human resources development and strengthening of managerial systems.[143]

The fundamental goal of capacity building is to enhance the ability to evaluate and address the crucial questions related to policy choices and modes of implementation among development options, based on an understanding of environment potentials and limits and of needs perceived by the people of the country concerned. It encompasses the country's human, scientific, technological, organizational, institutional and resource capabilities.[144]

Any capacity building programme will therefore be specific to regions and countries, but should also provide for global learning between regions. For vaccine safety communication, it should be integrated with other capacity building conducted by countries for immunization strengthening as well as for pharmacovigilance, and public health and regulatory system strengthening.

---

[142] Network for Education and Support in Immunisation (NESI). Accessible at: http://www.nesi.be/about-us/about-us.

[143] United Nations Development Programme (UNDP). UNDP Briefing Paper. New York: UNDP, 1991.

[144] United Nations Conference on Environment and Development (UNCED). Capacity building. In: UNCED. Agenda 21, Rio de Janeiro: UNCED, 1992: Chapter 37.

ANNEX 1:
READING LIST

Below is a list of official guidance documents, major reports and scientific journal publications for reading and gaining further knowledge on specific aspects relevant to vaccine safety communication systems. This short list is provided in addition to the broader literature referenced in the footnotes of this report.

Vaccine risk communication

US Institute of Medicine, Vaccine Safety Forum. Risk communication and vaccination: summary of a workshop. Washington, DC: National Academy Press, 1997. Accessible at: https://www.nap.edu/catalog/5861/risk-communication-and-vaccination-workshop-summary.

World Health Organization Regional Office for Europe (WHO-EURO). Vaccination and Trust. How concerns arise and the role of communication in mitigating crises. Copenhagen: WHO-EURO; 2017. Accessible at: http://www.euro.who.int/en/health-topics/disease-prevention/vaccines-and-immunization/publications/2017/vaccination-and-trust-2017.

World Health Organization Regional Office for Europe (WHO-EURO). Vaccination and trust library. Copenhagen: WHO-EURO, 2017. Accessible at: http://www.euro.who.int/en/health-topics/disease-prevention/vaccines-and-immunization/publications/vaccination-and-trust.

WHO Collaborating Centre (WHO-CC) for Advocacy & Training in Pharmacovigilance. Vaccine pharmacovigilance toolkit. Accra: WHO-CC for Advocacy & Training in Pharmacovigilance, 2013. Accessible at: http://vaccinepvtoolkit.org.

European Medicines Agency (EMA) and Heads of Medicines Agencies. Guideline on good pharmacovigilance practices – product- or population-specific considerations I: vaccines for prophylaxis against infectious diseases. London: EMA, 2013. Accessible at: http://www.ema.europa.eu/ema/index.jsp?curl=pages/regulation/document_listing/document_listing_000345.jsp&mid=WC0b01ac058058f32c.

Accelerated Development of Vaccine beNefit-risk Collaboration in Europe (ADVANCE). Developing Communication Strategies on Vaccine Benefits and Risks. ADVANCE, 2017. Accessible at: http://www.advance-vaccines.eu/?page=publications&id=DELIVERABLES.

Larson H. The globalization of risk and risk perception: why we need a new model of risk communication for vaccines. Drug Saf. 2012, 35: 1053-1059.

Vaccine hesitancy

World Health Organization Regional Office for Europe (WHO-EURO). Guide to Tailoring Immunization Programmes. Copenhagen: WHO-EURO; 2013. Accessible at: http://www.euro.who.int/en/health-topics/disease-prevention/vaccines-and-immunization/activities/tailoring-immunization-programmes-to-reach-underserved-groups-the-tip-approach.

Jarret C, Wilson R, O'Leary M, Eckersberger E, Larson HJ; SAGE Working Group on Vaccine Hesitancy. Strategies for addressing vaccine hesitancy: a systematic review. Vaccine 2015; 33: 4180-4190.

Schuster M, Duclos P, eds. WHO Recommendations Regarding Vaccine Hesitancy. Vaccine [special edition]. 2015, 33 (34): 4155-4218. Accessible at: http://www.sciencedirect.com/science/journal/0264410X/33/34.

Peretti-Watel P, Larson HJ, Ward JK, Schulz WS, and Verger P. Vaccine hesitancy: clarifying a theoretical framework for an ambiguous notion. PLOS Currents Outbreaks, 2015 Feb 25. Edition 1.

Larson HJ, Jarret C, Eckersberger E, Smith DM, Paterson P. Understanding vaccine hesitancy around vaccines and vaccination from a global perspective: a systematic review of published literature, 2007-2012.

Vaccination trust-building

World Health Organization Regional Office for Europe (WHO-EURO). Vaccination and trust: How concerns arise and the role of communication in mitigating crises. Copenhagen, Denmark: WHO-EURO, 2017. Accessible at: http://www.euro.who.int/__data/assets/pdf_file/0004/329647/Vaccines-and-trust.PDF?ua=1

World Health Organization Regional Office for Europe (WHO-EURO). Vaccination and trust library. Copenhagen, Denmark: WHO-EURO, 2017. Accessible at: http://www.euro.who.int/en/health-topics/disease-prevention/vaccines-and-immunization/publications/vaccination-and-trust.

United Nations Children's Fund (UNICEF) Regional Office for South Asia. Building trust and responding to adverse events following immunisation in South Asia. Kathmandu: UNICEF South Asia, 2005. Accessible at: http://www.unicef.org/rosa/Immunisation_report_17May_05(final_editing_text).pdf.

European Centre for Disease Prevention and Control (ECDC). Communication on immunisation: building trust. Stockholm: ECDC, 2012. Accessible at: http://ecdc.europa.eu/en/publications/Publications/TER-Immunisation-and-trust.pdf.

United Nations Children's Fund (UNICEF). Building trust in immunization: partnering with religious leaders and groups. New York: UNICEF; 2004. Available at: https://www.unicef.org/publications/index_20944.html.

Risk perception and communication

Bennett P, Calman K, Curtis S, Smith D. Risk Communication and Public Health. 2nd ed. Oxford: Oxfird University presss; 2010.

Kasperson RE, Renn O, Slovic P, Brown HS, Emel J, Goble R, et al. The social amplification of risk: a conceptual framework. Risk Analysis. 1988, 8: 177-187.

Morgan MG, Fischhoff B, Bostrom A, Atman CJ. Risk communication: a mental models approach. Cambridge: Cambridge University Press, 2002.

Slovic P. The feeling of risk: new perspectives on risk perception. London, Washington DC: Earthscan, 2010.

Health communication and health literacy

Rimal RN, Lapinski MK. Why health communication is important in public health. Bulletin of WHO. 2009, 87: 247-247. Accessible at: http://www.who.int/bulletin/volumes/87/4/08-056713/en/.

US Centres for Disease Control and Prevention (CDC). Health communication and social marketing. Atlanta: CDC, 2014. Accessible at: https://www.thecommunityguide.org/sites/default/files/assets/What-Works-Health-Communication-factsheet-and-insert.pdf.

US Centres for Disease Control and Prevention (CDC). Health literacy [webpage]. Atlanta: CDC, 2016. Accessible at: https://www.cdc.gov/healthliteracy/basics.html.

Waisbord S, Larson H. Why invest in communication for immunization: evidence and lessons learned. Baltimore, New York: Health Communication Partnership based at Johns Hopkins Bloomberg School of Public Health, Center for Communication Programs and the United Nations Children's Fund (UNICEF), 2005. Accessible at: http://www.who.int/immunization/hpv/communicate/why_invest_in_communication_for_immunization_unicef_healthcommunicationspartnership_path_usaid.pdf.

Strategic health communication

The Health Communication Capacity Collaborative. The P-process: five steps to strategic communication. Baltimore: Johns Hopkins Bloomberg School of Public Health Center for Communication Programs, 2003. Accessible at: http://www.who.int/immunization/hpv/communicate/the_new_p_process_jhuccp_2003.pdf.

O'Sullivan GA, Yonkler JA, Morgan W, Merritt AP. A field guide to designing a health communication strategy. Baltimore, MD: Johns Hopkins Bloomberg School of Public Health, Center for Communication Programs: March 2003. Accessible at: http://ccp.jhu.edu/documents/A%20Field%20Guide%20to%20Designing%20Health%20Comm%20Strategy.pdf.

Minister of Health Canada. Strategic risk communications framework for Health Canada and the Public Health Agency of Canada. Ottawa: Minister of Health Canada, 2007. Accessible at: https://www.canada.ca/en/health-canada/corporate/about-health-canada/activities-responsibilities/risk-communications.html.

Fischhoff B, Brewer NT, Downs JS. Communicating risks and benefits: an evidence-based user's guide. Silver Spring: US Food and Drug Administration, 2009. Accessible at: http://www.fda.gov/downloads/AboutFDA/ReportsManualsForms/Reports/UCM268069.pdf.

Bahri P. Public pharmacovigilance communication: a process calling for evidence-based, objective-driven strategies. Drug Saf. 2010, 33: 1065-1079.

Development of communication materials

US Centres for Disease Control and Prevention (CDC). CDC clear communication index. Atlanta: CDC, 2014. Accessible at: http://www.cdc.gov/ccindex/.

Nelson DE. Communicating public health information effectively: a guide for practitioners. Washington, DC: American Public Health Association, 2002.

Hugman B. Healthcare communication. London: Pharmaceutical Press, 2013.

Health information technology

U.S. Department of Health and Human Services (HHS). Health communication and health information technology [webpage]. Washington, DC: HHS, 2017. Accessible at: https://www.healthypeople.gov/2020/topics-objectives/topic/health-communication-and-health-information-technology.

Interacting with the news media and social media

World Health Organization Regional Office for Europe (WHO-EURO). Vaccine safety events: managing the communications response. Copenhagen: WHO-EURO, 2013. Accessible at: http://www.euro.who.int/en/health-topics/communicable-diseases/influenza/publications/2013/vaccine-safety-events-managing-the-communications-response.

US Centres for Disease Control and Prevention (CDC). Health communicator's social media toolkit. Atlanta: CDC, 2011. Accessible at: http://www.cdc.gov/healthcommunication/toolstemplates/socialmediatoolkit_bm.pdf.

US Centres for Disease Control and Prevention (CDC). CDC's guide to writing for social media. Atlanta: CDC, 2012. Accessible at: http://www.cdc.gov/socialmedia/tools/guidelines/pdf/GuidetoWritingforSocialMedia.pdf.

Interactions between regulatory authorities and patient/consumer and healthcare professional organizations

European Medicines Agency (EMA). Revised framework for interaction between the European Medicines Agency and patients and consumers and their organisations. London: EMA, 2014. Accessible at: http://www.ema.europa.eu/docs/en_GB/document_library/Other/2009/12/WC500018013.pdf.

European Medicines Agency (EMA). Revised framework for interaction between the European Medicines Agency and healthcare professionals and their organisations. London: EMA, 2016. Accessible at: http://www.ema.europa.eu/docs/en_GB/document_library/Other/2016/12/WC500218303.pdf.

Crisis management and communication

Hugman B. Expecting the worst. Uppsala: Uppsala Monitoring Centre, 2010. Extract accessible at: http://vaccinepvtoolkit.org/pv-toolkit/communication-and-crisis-management-in-vaccine-pharmacovigilance/#tab-id-1.

World Health Organization Regional Office for Europe (WHO-EURO). Vaccine safety events: managing the communications response. Copenhagen: WHO-EURO, 2013. Accessible at: http://www.euro.who.int/en/health-topics/communicable-diseases/influenza/publications/2013/vaccine-safety-events-managing-the-communications-response.

Capacity-building

Public Health Agency of Canada. Core competencies for public health in Canada. Ottawa: Public Health Agency of Canada, 2008. Accessible at: http://www.phac-aspc.gc.ca/php-psp/ccph-cesp/pdfs/cc-manual-eng090407.pdf.

ANNEX 2:
CONTRIBUTION TO THE CIOMS GUIDE TO ACTIVE VACCINE SAFETY SURVEILLANCE

Communication for active surveillance studies[145]

A major part of conducting a study is communicating with all involved parties and the general public, including the media. Communicating is likewise crucial for those authorizing and overseeing the study conduct. It is crucial to communicate with policy-makers, including legislators and politicians, to ensure continued support from national authorities for well-designed studies. The communication process should commence early, when designing the study and obtaining ethical and community approval prior to its start. Clarity and common agreement on the study objectives is key in this respect.

Communication requires setting up a network and mechanisms for multi-party interactions and in particular exchange with the concerned communities, as well as maintaining these interactions throughout the study process. Listening is an essential part of communication, a key component which promotes understanding. Listening should address questions or concerns raised by the concerned communities and stakeholders, both proactively in the protocol and during the conduct of the study.

Communication materials, such as informed consent forms, should be adapted to the target audience in their information content, presentation and tone. Experience has shown that objectives, risks and ethical standards of studies can be questioned from inside and outside the concerned communities, even when a study is already ongoing. Without continuous preparedness and responsiveness of the communication system at any point in time, this may lead to a crisis of trust and premature ending of a study to the disadvantage of individual and community health. This may happen when an AEFI occurs or a new risk is identified, but also due to other concerns of the public.

The practical aspects of conducting studies described below mention at which stages communication becomes particularly important. A specific section gives recommendations for communicating study findings. The fundamental guiding principle for communication is honesty about expected benefits, risks and uncertainties. Persons in charge of communication should be well trained and approach these activities in an alert, empathetic and professional manner.

Communication of study findings

The recommendations for communication for active surveillance studies above should be applied for communicating the study findings. The objectives of this part of the communication process are to provide information about the safety and benefit-risk balance, in order to support decision-making for immunization policies and individual informed choice in relation to immunization, and to support the safe and effective use of vaccines. Best communication practices, developed by the health communication sciences, for lingual, numerical and visual expression of the findings should be followed. The public also needs to receive explanations on the study rationale and be enabled to

---

[145] Council for International Organizations of Medical Sciences (CIOMS). CIOMS Guide to Active Vaccine Safety Surveillance (report of the CIOMS Working Group on Vaccine Safety). Geneva: CIOMS, 2017, Chapter 4, section 4.1 Communication for the conduct of AVSS, p.45 and section 4.6 Communication of study findings, p.54.

understand the robustness and the credibility of the data and their analysis, including the trustworthiness of those having conducted and overseen the study. This requires an in-depth understanding of the knowledge and sentiments prevalent in the public and pre-testing of information materials for assuring that they meet the communication objectives. A media conference should be considered to present the results and answer questions. The wider dissemination of the study results should reach those who need to know. Contact points for questions from the public should be in place.

ANNEX 3:
MEMBERSHIP, EXTERNAL REVIEWERS, AND MEETINGS

The CIOMS Working Group on Vaccine Safety (WG) was formed in 2013 following the completion of CIOMS/WHO Working Group on Vaccine Pharmacovigilance to continue addressing unmet needs in the area of vaccine pharmacovigilance and specifically address Objective #8 of WHO's Global Vaccine Safety Initiative regarding public-private information exchange. The original composition of the group consisted of experts from regulatory, public health, academia, and industry.

The WG met in a series of eight meetings from May 2013 through March 2016. Some representatives changed during the years according to organizational and professional developments.

The seven members of the Editorial Team on the CIOMS Guide to Active vaccine safety surveillance were: Steven R. Bailey (Editor-in-Chief), Novilia Bachtiar, Irina Caplanusi, Frank DeStefano, Corinne Jouquelet-Royer, Paulo Santos, and Patrick Zuber. CIOMS staff and advisors who supported this WG include: Lembit Rägo, Gunilla Sjölin-Forsberg, Ulf Bergman, Karin Holm (Technical Collaboration Coordinator and CIOMS In-house Editor), Amanda Owden, and Sue le Roux.

The WG developed into three main topic groups (TG) with associated deliverables and leaders as follows:

Topic Group	Deliverable	Leadership
TG1 on Essential Vaccine Information (Appendix I of the Guide to AVSS) -	Appendix I of CIOMS Guide to AVSS	Ulrich Heininger (final stage) David Martin (early stage)
TG2 on Active Vaccine Safety Surveillance	CIOMS Guide to AVSS (Steven Bailey, WG Editor-in-Chief)	Steven Bailey, Mimi Darko, Corinne Jouquelet-Royer (final stage) Françoise Sillan (early stage)
TG3 on Vaccine Safety Communication	CIOMS Guide to Vaccine Safety Communication (Priya Bahri, Editor)	Priya Bahri (final stage) Ken Hartigan-Go (first stage) Felix Arellano (initial stage)

During the course of its work, topic group 3 evolved in its focus. Its genesis started from the first WG meeting in London when vaccine crisis management arose as an area needing greater public-private interaction, with Felix Arellano serving as topic group leader initially. When he later changed affiliations, Ken Hartigan-Go assumed leadership and broadened the scope of the topic group. Subsequently, Hartigan-Go passed leadership to Priya Bahri who stepped in to lead the topic group in late 2015 and forged a new direction based on member and broader stakeholder input.

The table below shows a cumulative list of WG members who have been important contributors to TG3 on communication over the last four years, organized alphabetically by last name, and their associated organizations. These contributors have served as members or alternates in the Working Group for differing periods of time; some have contributed for the full duration (2013 to 2017), while others have attended at least one meeting and/or contributed to TG3's development. In some cases organizations changed names over the course of this project or contributors changed affiliations; this is not always reflected in the listing. The list generally includes the affiliation of the contributor during the time he or she participated in the topic group. Unless indicated otherwise the comments from external reviewers were considered as expert, personal opinions and not necessarily representing those of their employers or affiliations.

CIOMS Working Group on Vaccine Safety -- Topic Group 3 on Vaccine Safety Communication – Active members and affiliations

	WG Member Name	Organization (Stakeholder group)
1.	Abdoellah, Siti Asfijah	Indonesia National Agency of Drug and Food Control (Regulatory authority)
2.	Arellano, Felix	Merck (Pharma industry)
3.	Bachtiar, Novilia	Bio Farma Indonesia (Pharma industry)
4.	Bahri, Priya	European Medicines Agency (Regulatory authority)
5.	Bergman, Ulf	Council for International Organizations of Medical Sciences (CIOMS, Senior Adviser)
6.	Chandler, Rebecca	Uppsala Monitoring Centre (Independent foundation and WHO Collaborating Centre)
7.	Chua, Peter Glen	Philippines FDA (Regulatory authority)
8.	Darko, Mimi Delese	Ghana Food and Drug Authority (Regulatory authority)
9.	Dodoo, Alexander	University of Ghana (Academia) and WHO Collaborating Centre for Advocacy and Training in Pharmacovigilance
10.	Hartigan-Go, Ken	Philippines Dept of Health (Public health authority), Asian Institute of Management
11.	Lindquist, Marie	Uppsala Monitoring Centre (Independent foundation and WHO Collaborating Centre)
12.	Santos, Paulo	Bio-Manguinhos / Fiocruz (Government pharma)
13.	Zuber, Patrick	World Health Organization (U.N. specialized agency for health)

CIOMS Working Group on Vaccine Safety meetings*

	Date	Location	Host
1.	May 2013	London, UK	European Medicines Agency
2.	September 2013	Geneva, Switzerland	World Health Organization
3.	February 2014	Atlanta, Georgia, USA	Centers for Disease Control and Prevention

	Date	Location	Host
4.	May 2014	Uppsala, Sweden	Uppsala Monitoring Centre
5.	September 2014	Rabat, Morocco	Centre d'Antipoison et Pharmacovigilance de Maroc
6.	May 2015	Lyon, France	Sanofi Pasteur
7.	September 2015	Collegeville, near Philadelphia, Pennsylvania, USA	Pfizer
8.	March 2016	Accra, Ghana	Ghana Food and Drug Authority

* Costs for travel to face-to-face meetings and accommodation were covered by each Working Group member's parent organization *or by CIOMS as per rules*, and were not covered by the meeting hosts. Numerous virtual meetings by teleconference were arranged and covered both by CIOMS as well as by member organizations.

The editors solicited feedback from outside experts and WHO staff for the later drafts. During the public consultation via the CIOMS website from 28 August to 11 October 2017, comments were received from experienced institutions and public health/vaccine communication experts. Their comments were welcoming and supportive to the report, and clarifications on the recommendations and updates to some of the references, as well as additions to the reading list have been implemented in the final report in response to the comments. CIOMS thanks those who commented for their time and support.

CIOMS Working Group on Vaccine Safety -- Vaccine Safety Communication – External contributors, reviewers, and public consultation

	Name	Organization
1.	Bruce Hugman	Uppsala Monitoring Centre, Sweden
2.	Katrine Bach Habersaat	WHO Regional Office for Europe, Copenhagen, Denmark
3.	Patrick Zuber	WHO Vaccine Safety
4.	Madhav Ram Balakrishnan	WHO Vaccine Safety
5.	Heidi Larson	London School of Hygiene & Tropical Medicine, UK (during public consultation commented in private capacity)
6.	Jeanet Kemmeren	National Institute for Public Health and the Environment (Netherlands) (during public consultation commented for the organization)

	Name	Organization
7.	Julia Tainijoki-Seyer	World Medical Association (during public consultation commented for the organization)
8.	Robert Pless	Health Canada (during public consultation commented in private capacity)
9.	Steve Anderson	U.S. Food and Drug Administration, Office of Biostatistics and Epidemiology, CBER (during public consultation commented for the organization)